COMMONSENSE SEX

COMMONSENSE SEX

SEX

*   *   *

A BASIS
FOR DISCUSSION
AND REAPPRAISAL

*

by Ronald Michael Mazur

BEACON PRESS

Boston

Copyright © 1968 by Ronald Michael Mazur
Library of Congress catalog card number: 68–27521
International Standard Book Number: 0–8070–2797–9
First published as a Beacon Paperback in 1973
Beacon Press books are published under the auspices
of the Unitarian Universalist Association
Published simultaneously in Canada
by Saunders of Toronto, Ltd.
All rights reserved
Printed in the United States of America

Dedicated to

DAUGHTER, MICHAL
SON, NATHAN
AND THEIR GENERATION

Contents

Contents

Acknowledgments

I am grateful to Peter A. Bertocci, Borden P. Bowne Professor of Philosophy, Boston University, for his rare ability to awaken students from "dogmatic slumber"; to James Luther Adams, Mallinkrodt Professor of Divinity, Harvard Divinity School, for translating ethics from dusty tomes into inspiration for action; to Lester Dearborn, pioneer sexologist and marriage counselor, for his leadership of the Clergy for the Advancement of Sex Education; and to Harry C. Meserve, editor of the *Journal of Religion and Health*, and Graham B. Blaine, Jr., Chief of Psychiatric Services, Harvard University, for their encouragement of a research proposal to the Academy of Religion and Mental Health which led me into serious involvement with this book's subject.

May all wise scholars and teachers be spared blame for the work of their disciples.

For the existence of the book, I thank: John Huenefeld of Beacon Press, for pressing conversation into writing; my wife, Joyce, for valuable suggestions about content; and Mrs. Anne Bullard, my secretary, who patiently transformed scribbles into manuscript.

A Personal Word to the Reader

THERE IS A DEGREE OF PRE-sumptuousness on the part of an author who attempts to share personal convictions, concerns, attitudes, and values about essential aspects of sex and sexuality. Yet, as difficult as it is to present clearly my honest thoughts on the subject with the goal of stimulating your own thinking, it is even more difficult to remain silent. Our age is straddling the threshold of a new era of enlightened, healthy, and responsible sexual emancipation, and the time is overdue for forthright consideration of the subject from those involved with institutionalized religion. Too, I feel an urgency for a more rapid evolution of sane social expectations concerning sexual behavior as I continually stand helplessly by and watch so many people needlessly torturing their consciences, warping their growth, and damaging their lives because of the contemporary dilemma in man-woman relationships. Understand, please, that I do not have definite answers to these complex problems which beset us all. It is simply that in striving to understand myself, to work with my wife for a creative marriage, to provide helpful guidelines for my children, and to minister effectively to the basic human problems of my parishioners, I find it necessary to clarify and articulate my framework for making some sense out of all the problems and questions surrounding this vital dimension of life.

I propose to put on the line my reflections for your consideration, not with the intention of convincing you to adopt them, but with the earnest hope that, by testing your ideas against mine, you will determine for yourself an approach to sex which will do justice to your fullest potential as a person. Your answers for yourself, in accordance with your beliefs and ideals, may very well differ from mine. Although this book is offered primarily to unmarried young adults, it contains material relevant to everyone and can provide a ground for dialogue between generations. Most importantly, what is herein presented fills the sizeable gap between childhood sex education and the information of marriage manuals. What we seem incapable of accepting in our society is that young and not-so-young unmarried persons participate in a variety of sexual dilemmas and experiences. Adults and parents are, of course, much more comfortable when preaching to youth about the glories of marriage and the miracle of babies, but this approach ignores the condition and needs of single people who have no intention of jumping prematurely into marriage. We should face the fact that sex is separable not only from procreation but from the state of matrimony.

This book is entitled *Commonsense Sex*. What is common may not make sense, and what is sensible may not be common. And certainly, in the area of sex standards and behavior what is sensible to one may be sensational to another. However, it is my assumption that even the sensitive and sensible person in high school is able to reason about such matters without benefit of advanced learning in theology, philosophy, or psychology. These academic disciplines obviously have a great deal to teach us, and, as a matter of fact, we all operate with theological, philosophical, and psychological presuppositions even though not trained to conceptualize them. I speak here as plainly and forthrightly as possible without appeal to any particular school of thought, leaving it open for you to ask at every turn, "Does this make sense to me?" and then to determine your own answers within your own frames of reference. The commonsense approach is exemplified to me by the little boy who, in the midst of a gullible and subservient crowd, exclaimed, as the emperor went by in regal procession, "But he has nothing on!" Perhaps, with such childlike honesty and directness we can look together at sexual practices clothed with custom and perceive the bareness and embarrassment of present-day sexual illusions.

Ronald Michael Mazur
SALEM, MASSACHUSETTS
APRIL 15, 1968

COMMONSENSE SEX

Education for Love: The Wider Context of Sex Education

THIS BOOK OF OPINIONS CON-
cerning contemporary sexual relationships, addressed primarily
to unmarried young adults, is not a book about "sex education" as that term is popularly understood. There is very little
information here pertaining to the physiology, biology, and
chemistry of sex. Rather the focus is on the philosophy, psychology, and morality of human relations which are, by definition, sexual in nature. Sex is given to us and is not in and of
itself a problem; sexuality is learned, and therein lies our
dilemma. You were born a male or a female and can procreate
without difficulty, but only with difficulty can you learn to be
a man or woman who can create.

Please understand at the outset: It is not that there is
little to learn about the physical functions of sex. On the
contrary, there is much to learn; yet, it is only within the last
few years that there has been any significant attempt to bring
into our schools the available knowledge about humans as
sexual beings.

We have long proclaimed that the proper study of mankind is man, but we have conveniently ignored the obvious
fact that man is composed of men and women, of males and
females. Quite generally, the approach to education about
sex is pathetic. We gingerly seek to introduce courses on the
high-school level, even while we realize that the subject ought
to be introduced in kindergarten and incorporated systemati-

cally into grades one through six so that by the time children reach the age of twelve, they are familiar with the essential facts of reproduction and human anatomy.

Nevertheless, there are encouraging signs. Professional societies focusing upon the subject are forming; good textbooks and curricula are being written; and state public school systems, national private school associations, and major religious educational resources are mobilizing to correct the situation. The combined educational endeavor of all such agencies, plus the increasing availability of safe and simple chemical contraceptives, will soon bring our culture to the stage of enlightenment in matters of sex information and knowledge.

What concerns educators in several fields is that understanding about sexuality must accompany knowledge about sex. It is, for example, one thing to know about contraceptives, but it is a different thing to understand how sexual intimacy affects human relationships. It is one thing to be free of the old taboos; it is yet another matter to understand how to use this freedom to enhance the integrity of your partner and yourself. Our culture is finally removing the veil from sex knowledge, but most educational institutions are still pretty squeamish about facing forthrightly the inevitably changing patterns of sexual behavior and the attendant value and attitudinal changes which must be shaped in the younger generation. For the most part, young adults are going it alone without honest guidelines from parents, teachers, and clergy.

This irresponsibility on the part of the older generation leaves contemporary youth open to victimization of commercial sex. The communications media relentlessly exploit ignorance, anxieties, and gullibility, and feed us a steady diet of sentimental slop. The old stereotypes of "maleness" and "femaleness" still distort our image of ourselves and our expectations of others. But the common sense of the younger generation is evident in the widespread revolt against the old wives' tales, the old clichés, and the romantic notions of a bygone era. It is currently fashionable to doubt that we are engaged in a genuine sexual revolution. It is often said, for instance, that people have always done what is now being done, and the only difference is that now our behavior is more open and our expressed values are catching up with our formerly hidden behavior. And, of course, there is much truth to the assertion that what we are now witnessing is a climactic phase of an evolution toward sexual freedom. Nevertheless, the term "revolution" best expresses the nature of the contemporary changes in patterns of sexual conduct and conviction.

The Essence of the Sexual Revolution

Underlying the following discussion of the sexual revolution are two primary factors known as "the pill" and "the new morality" which will be considered in Chapters 7 and 10 respectively. The developments explored here are not new in themselves, and can be traced through many authors and innumerable sociological changes spanning hundreds of years. But, taken together, they have the impact of shaping a new human condition which must be faced with new attitudes and approaches. We are past the point where "the old morality" (or traditional social norms) can merely be patched up with inventive exhortations and eloquent appeals to the "faith of our fathers."

The Personal Nature of Intimate Relationships Once it was widely assumed that the "good" kids could be distinguished from the "bad" kids. What panics the older generation is that such simple distinctions no longer apply. Parents are shocked to discover, for instance, that their "good" kids spend weekends in bed with their lovers or that they set up house off campus without the sanction of a marriage license. Obviously, the overwhelming majority of young adults do not express their independence by such extremes of sexual freedom. Yet, no matter how outwardly conventional they are, by choice or by chance, their reactions to such things are quite different from those of their parents, teachers, and religious leaders. They may not agree with such independence but they are not shocked, and, given the opportunity, they would consider participating in such behavior more seriously than their parents would ever realize. Basically, the question confronting young adults today is not, "To bed or not to bed?" but rather "To bed with whom and under what conditions?" At the very least, they face the "problems" of petting with greater poise and with less shame than did the teenager of a generation ago.

The widespread assumption that "immorality" is rampant in the younger generation is unfortunate. It is not realized that youth is searching for higher levels of integrity and honesty, and that there is a tender trust and depth of loveliness in their intimate relationships which is a tribute to humanity. This is not to imply that all young adults have only wisdom, maturity, and pure, unmixed motives. But, generally speaking, much of the unconventional moral behavior which exists is of high character.

What it comes to is this: "Father and Mother, I don't intend to hurt you, but I must risk finding my own way in a society which constantly preaches love but which does not exemplify it or know what it is all about." Such firm insistence upon the right of the individual to explore taboo territory and to make personal judgment upon personal relationships is a relatively new phenomenon in our society. More young adults than ever before are taking this right and this risk, and those who exercise this responsibility are also learning the hazards involved—learning which contributes to both personal growth and to the fashioning of a saner society.

The Humanization of the Sexes   Perhaps the most far-reaching change which has crystalized in our evolution is the realization that both males and females are persons: human beings with similar desires, needs, and goals. We are finally reaching the point of going beyond the old arguments as to the proper social roles for men versus women. The battle of the sexes is now giving way to the war between the dehumanizers and the humanizers. The folly of forcing persons into traditional social roles and functions simply on the basis of sex is now recognized. The old categories of "masculinity" and "femininity" have happily broken down in large measure, and, while we will *forever* have spirited controversy about the nature of man vis-à-vis woman, we have expanded marvelously the freedom of the individual to become what he (she) needs and wants to be regardless of sex. The old definitions of "manhood" and "womanhood" served the purpose of their times, but we are faced with the challenge of formulating new definitions for our time.

More specifically, this challenge boils down to the old phenomenon of the "double standard": One set of rules, expectations, and privileges for men, and another for women. This phenomenon has forever helped and plagued mankind and it is a virtue of our times that we are confronting it and seeking solutions openly. The question of the double standard involves the issues of virginity and the meanings of love, which are dealt with in Chapters 6 and 3 respectively. It will suffice to say now that young people are doing a tremendous job in demolishing the insidious aspects of male dominance and egocentricity as it is reflected in the double standard. And, fortunately, men are also assisting in this assault upon their time-honored prerogatives of "seed sowing." Men have had to pretend that they were lustier and more "sexy." Consequently, they have forced themselves into absurd models and expectations of "virility" and "masculinity" which they cannot live up to and which actually destroy their fuller potential as sensitive and loving members of the human race. The quality of human life suffers because of the tragic number of boys who think that they must "conquer" a girl before they can become men, and because of the overwhelming number of girls who think they must suppress their sexual satisfaction in order to be acceptable marriage material (discount for the moment the girls who use sex to snare husbands, because this technique requires the double standard in order to operate). People raised in the old-school conceptions of sex lament the diffusion of sex roles, but the so-called feminization of the male and the so-called masculinization of the female is a healthy indication that everybody is becoming more human.

The younger generation is caught in this process of the humanization of the sexes, but it is a "breakthrough" generation and it will be to its credit that it persevered in the quest for sexual equality in spite of the censures against it.

Our time is now single-standard time. Males no longer have alibis for sexual irresponsibility. The same holds true for females. The double standard is finally breaking down, not so much because men are more enlightened, but more because women no longer tolerate the terms of the man-woman game as defined by men.

The Enjoyment of Sexuality   Procreation as the prime function of sex has now receded into anthropological antiquity as the recreational aspects of it are more widely accepted and enjoyed. Obviously, casual sex is subject to commercial crassness as well as to interpersonal abuse, but unmarried young adults are today more inclined to use sex as a pleasant pastime without the absurd and hypocritical formality of the engagement period. Religious groups view with horror the divorce of sex from procreation, but it is a trend which was cut deeply into patterns of human behavior with the advent of contraceptive devices; and, now, with the availability of the pill, it is irreversible. It yet remains an awkward stage in the becoming of Man, but there is great promise for a happier human race.

The Contemporary Postsex Character of Sexuality

The three developments just mentioned, namely, the search for honest interpersonal encounter, the attention to the personal needs of both sexes, and the diminishing procreative function of sex, merge with force in our time to create the impact of a sexual revolution. And the essence of this revolution is that, in our culture, we are at the point of going beyond sex to sexuality. The old dilemmas, shames, guilts, prohibitions, and restrictions no longer form the framework of our problems, except insofar as they contribute to the "generation gap." Our understanding of our own sexuality and of man-woman relationships must be seen in a new perspective more relevant for us and our children. Genital sex is giving way to congenial sexuality. As sane sexual freedom increases, we will be less possessed by the desires for a "lay" and more sensitive to the quality of our intimate relationships.

Already, there is a wider context of sex education to concern us. For as we gradually learn to accept the simple reality and loveliness of sex and its delights and functions, we face the more important question of the attitudes and interpersonal values necessary to live with and live up to. It is not enough to know how to make love; we must learn how to be loving.

CHAPTER 2

The Shame of Shame

MOST OF US STRIVE FOR SIGNS of approval. We need acceptance and praise from others; we strive to conform to the particular expectations and norms of the groups within which we circulate or to which we would like to gain entrance. However, far too many of the worries and tribulations which beset us are unnecessary because they stem not from originating or internal goals, but from copying or external authorities—authorities which shame us into compliance. Convention and authority are admittedly indispensable forces shaping our lives. Furthermore, such forces can be and often are constructive. But this same socialization process which enfolds us from birth can be a warping influence as well, and sometimes we can pay much too high a price for being "nice" or "good" in conventional terms.

The Dilemma of Growing Up By the time we are young adults we are accomplished in the act of hiding our selfhood, indeed, the socialization process can be so efficient that we may not even be conscious of a deep inner need for self-actualization. We simply form patterns of reaction to the demands and expectations of parents, school, friends, and religious institutions; therefore, if the resulting personality package is attractive, receives attention, or just gets us by, we experience little agony of self-appraisal and go on about the normal business of doing what is expected. While we are young we are so involved in, and pressured by, the conventional standards of success and so involved in testing ourselves against the goading demands of society that we have not enough time, experience, or education to consider more significant alternatives for our lives. True, in any generation there is that minor percentage of young adults who are social renegades, who do not do what is expected because they sense that the road laid out for them leads nowhere in terms of the ideals and values they conscientiously hold.

Unfortunately, it is not until "middlessence" that the vast majority of men and women will be overwhelmed with feelings of emptiness or meaninglessness, wondering who they are, what they want, and where they want to go. Some people will break under the stress of such identity, value, or professional crises; some will simply sink into the sadness of "quiet desperation"; some will panic and try all sorts of things in order to make life entertaining or exciting. At this middle-aged stage of life most people are restless without direction and inwardly miserable; they are comfortable with relatively good health and with a fair measure of material goods, but they have been trapped inside conventional molds and feel self-less. This condition is "normalcy" for millions and a menace to the well-being of the human race, for, as innocuous as this condition of unhappiness sounds, it leads to self-hate, bitterness, and impulses for destruction. Emotional sickness of all kinds is bred of despair, and there is neither kindness nor understanding of others where there is no respect and knowledge of the self. Unhappy individuals are happiest when they are consoling others, and those who are basically insecure feel big when stepping on others, usually in the name of some ideology or noble cause. Those who cannot live freely will not let live.

The Scars of Shame   Shaming is the insidious technique of conformity. An authoritarian personality resorts to shaming because its power does not rest on reasonable persuasion but on exploiting the submissiveness of shaky individuals who cannot afford ridicule. "Shame on you!" is an insult that sears the soul in infancy and remains an eternal echo in the self, crushing us time and time again with irrational feelings of inferiority. Think for a moment of how often days are ruined with moods of anger, resentment, or vague feelings of helplessness or apology. Somebody is always making us feel foolish or at least trying to do so. It seems as if for the first twenty-five years of our lives, if not longer, we are constantly answerable to somebody for everything we do, or want to do, or even for what we think. And unless we are blessed with wise and loving parents and teachers, our education may sometimes be at the expense of our dignity. Learning mistakes are often not permitted; parent and teacher pounce on ignorance and use that occasion of correction for shallow self-esteem. This also happens in other areas of learning and in all the one-upmanship games people play. True, most of these encounters are not traumatic for us; we often are not conscious of them. There is even a trial by shame through which we have to survive for close relationships with others. When we are new on a job, for example, we find that there is an initial testing time when our fellow workers put us through the ropes, but if we persevere with humor and our fallibility is clearly revealed to the satisfaction of all, we then become accepted. The same process seems to operate in the military, in college fraternities, in professional societies, and in neighborhood social circles. It would appear that others are more comfortable with our weaknesses than with our strengths.

There is value, however, in having to go through the fires of shaming attempts on the part of others, for this can be a strengthening experience by seeing the self in dramatic contrast to them. We are forced to find the courage to assert ourselves, to be more than passive or easily manipulated for the immature satisfaction of another. This critical lesson in life is often very painful and can crush some personalities into lifelong submission. This is why it is so important to allow youngsters to make their own mistakes, to aid them in gaining self-confidence and a sense of independence. Perhaps the two greatest character assets that any individual can develop are a sense of humor and a compassionate acceptance of every human being's idiosyncrasies and weaknesses. No person is perfect. We all make mistakes, and the chances for self-improvement are vastly increased when someone whom we respect helps us to face ourselves and to desire self-change.

For the sake of our wholeness it is imperative to grow beyond shame. We can learn from this kind of experience—it is almost inevitable—but we must realize that we have been bludgeoned with the crude tools of the socialization process, and ought to persevere in developing the attitudes and the values which will help us become unshameable.

Shame Versus Guilt   The reason it is so difficult to become unshameable is that we confuse the feelings of shame with guilt. These feelings have a similar emotional impact: We suddenly find our integrity exposed and threatened by a judgment made against us. We feel embarrassed. One way to distinguish the difference between shame and guilt is to say that in shame we are embarrassed before men while in guilt we are embarrassed before God. Another way to indicate the difference is to say that shame is a feeling we have when noticed by others doing something *they* think is wrong, while guilt is a feeling we have when noticed by others or by ourselves in doing something *we* think is wrong. When we feel guilt we may also feel ashamed, but feeling shame does not necessarily mean that we feel guilt. Masturbation and "playing doctor" are perhaps classic examples of our confusion of shame with guilt and the lasting negative effects which such confusion can cause. For example, a child is enjoying self-stimulation—perhaps even absent-mindedly—when an adult enters and proclaims, "Don't!" with the same emotional urgency as if the child were leaning too far out of a rowboat. The consequence: "I'm bad," says the child to himself. When we are older it is to be hoped that we realize the inevitability and innocence of such child's play, but the adult's "Don't!" has been confused with a divine "Thou shalt not!" and the damage has been done: We continue to feel shame about nakedness and sensual pleasure.

Contemporary psychologists recognize that people develop emotional difficulties because they are unable to incorporate into their personalities an integral value system which frees them from the more or less arbitrary prohibitions of mores. Such integral value systems produce feelings of genuine guilt which are indispensable to the healthy person. Conscience is the feeling of "I ought" as opposed to the feeling of "You must." When we do not submit to the "You must" we feel shame; when we do not listen to our "I ought" we feel guilty.

Genuine guilt is a wonderful capability. It shows a conscience which is a vital dimension of the healthy, self-actualizing person. A person who has never achieved a conscience which can produce guilt suffers from the most serious character disorder possible.

The task of the moral person is to decrease his vulnerability to shame and to increase his sensitivity to guilt—and to know the difference.

Guilt and Sinfulness Distinguishing between shame and guilt is no easy task. At the risk of complicating the issue, let us consider shame and guilt in the context of the concept of sin even though various religions view it differently.

It is important to realize that for at least the past twenty-five years there has been a convergence of the disciplines of theology and psychiatry in their respective understandings of the "human condition." This literature is vast, complex, and technical. Contemporary theologians talk in terms of "estrangement" and psychologists talk about "alienation." Theologians use the concepts "redemption" or "reconciliation" and psychologists use "self-actualization" or "integrity." Both disciplines, though not in full agreement, are pointing toward the same human search for "wholeness of being."

A person usually thinks of sin in terms of the transgression of specific laws handed down to him in his tradition. The Ten Commandments, for example, have a central place in the religious ethic of most people. And sins are felt to be committed when these commandments are broken.

The new context for understanding sin, however, does not give a central place to traditional religious laws. This is not to say that these laws are scoffed at or held to be unimportant or inconsequential. On the contrary, these laws and traditions are considered valuable guidelines. The emphasis, however, is on the condition or state of being rather than on the mechanical or automatic obeying of rules or laws. For example, consider the commandment to "honor thy father and mother." Does this mean to do whatever your mother or father commands you to do? What if you are more morally sensitive than your mother and father? What do you do if, in conscience, you must do otherwise than that ordered by them? This commandment is good because it obligates children to follow the guidance of their parents. In the last analysis, however, you may have to conclude that in the light of your own understanding and situation, the expectations of your parents will compromise your own integrity. Such a confrontation can be very painful emotionally. Most of us want very much to conform to parental direction since parents make many sacrifices for our welfare. Nevertheless, in some situations, we may be obliged to follow our own conscientious direction, risking alienation from our parents when they cannot relate to us as individual persons. If we face such a choice, it is important that we differentiate shame from guilt in our own reactions. We may experience shame because of the social and religious pressures to conform to our parents' directives, but if we have been thoughtful and conscientious in our choice, we will not feel guilty.

An analogy can be made with reference to civil law. We recognize that law in democratic process is devised for the maximum well-being of all citizens. Civil law, however, by its very nature is caught in a "cultural lag": It applies to past social conditions rather than shaping present social conditions. When we demonstrate or protest against laws which we consider inequitable in the light of new opportunities for social progress, we may have to suffer legal consequences rather than stifle our consciences. The suffocation of the self is too high a price to pay for cultural conformity, especially when certain forms of conformity entail social injustice.

We can also lapse into a state of sinfulness, that is, betray our own integrity, by what we do *not* do as well as by what we do. The new understanding of guilt and shame takes seriously sins of omission and calls us beyond the legalism of the letter of the law to the spirit of the law. Committing sins is child's play in the sense that, as children, we need basic specific laws to shape our social and moral behavior and, sooner or later, we discover both our fallibility and freedom as we test the limits of such laws. As we mature we see that these elementary "do's" and "don't's" are themselves subject to interpretation and that they are inadequate guides in the face of complicated moral decisions. And so we do our best to make honest and worthwhile moral choices. Even if we make a poor choice, or see later that we were wrong, we can still be free of guilt. On the other hand, we may comply with the traditional, essential moral laws and have a constant nagging sense of guilt because we have been morally sloppy, have been afraid to risk difficult decisions, or have held back from making the extra effort that we could have made. Thus, though we may appear to be morally blameless according to anyone else's judgment, we may feel the condition of sinfulness because we are fragmented within ourselves and do not actively choose the highest good we know. And, the reverse is possible: Others may blame and shame us because of apparent sinful behavior, but, if our action is committed out of integrity we will not feel divided within ourselves and will not be emotionally crippled with guilt. Rather, we shall know a freedom of being which strengthens our internal resources, enabling us to make a more substantial contribution to life.

Life: A Matter of Living　　How can we avoid the trap of conventionalism and live to our fullest capacity a continuing love affair with life? Obviously, there is no easy answer. But there are some approaches to sustain us in the process of creative searching. At the outset it should be realized that the trials and tensions of growing up cannot be avoided; they are the warp and woof of human existence. Young people who want everything to "come up roses" throughout the adolescent phase of maturation will have to learn the hard way. When we are girls and boys we have the problems of girls and boys, and it is not until we are men and women that we understand as men and women. Do not misunderstand: Wisdom is not simply a product of aging. But there are phases or stages of growing, each with their respective problems which are felt by each person in a unique way. No one else can do our living for us, and no matter how sound the advice given us when we are young, we must each make our own peace with the inevitable dilemmas we will encounter. At best, we can be provided with helpful examples for living by authorities we can respect, and gain healthful attitudes and concepts which will sustain us when the going gets rough. And even if we are emotionally crippled by our upbringing, we may yet be sane enough to "break down" and begin again the process of maturing. This is the more painful route to wholeness of being, but it is worth every agony to dig away the emotional encrustations and make the exciting discovery of the self. Such persistence in the risky adventure of becoming more human is a tribute to the marvelous resiliency of the psyche and a testimony to the courage of countless men and women.

Parents do, of course, have their difficulties in applying the insights of adult experience to attitudes and behavior; they themselves are beset with their burden of shames. It seems easier to let unconventional thoughts and attitudes lie secret, remaining unexpressed even between husband and wife. It is also easier to allow one's children to be molded by social mores than to share with them honest feelings or doubts or to risk being thought of as "loose" parents if the children seem too sophisticated in matters sexual. It is probably good for the evolution of civilization for younger generations to be suspicious and scornful of society as a whole, but when it comes to judgmental mistrust of everyone over thirty, including one's parents, an impoverishing communication gap can be the only result. Adolescents may not want to be like the adults and socializing authorities who have raised them, and they may even be justified in their criticisms. But for the sake of sanity and wisdom it must be realized that older generations too have suffered through conditions not of their creation, that all generations have ancient dilemmas in common, and that each generation makes some contribution to the welfare of the human family.

As for recognizing and avoiding the traps of sexual conventionalism while you are an unmarried young adult, the soundest advice is to take your time before settling down in matrimony, rather than being shamed into it. Unfortunately, many people undertake such a serious commitment before they have developed enough emotional stability, inner direction, self-understanding, and worldly experience. Maturity is, of course, a relative matter: One person at seventeen may have greater knowledge, stronger character, and a more profound ability for interpersonal relationships than another person of thirty-five. In general, however, those who marry in their teens are courting difficulties which can be disastrous. Why does a woman begin to feel herself a failure when she reaches twenty-five and is still unmarried? Why is a man of twenty-nine suspected of being a queer if he is still a bachelor? Why the panic for early marriage? The reasons are many: Anxious parents who breathe a sigh of relief when the child is finally respectably married; young women afraid they might never snag their catch; young adults who need to prove their independence; or the misleading concept in romantic love that happiness can be found only through another. There are numerous other reasons, but much attention should also be paid to the facts that our sexual needs urge us not to wait too long for satisfaction, and that the young unmarried adult lives in a state of limbo, expected to act like an adult but given neither the full privileges nor responsibilities of adulthood which, ironically, can be purchased cheaply, yet very expensively, in the form of a marriage license. It is perhaps a tribute to the attractiveness of the marital state that so many young people eagerly seek this covenant with such a high spirit of excitement and adventure. Nevertheless, there are many benefits to resisting unashamedly the pressures of surrendering singlehood. The constant question-accusation, "Why aren't you married yet?" should be countered with the more intelligent question-response, "Why should I want to be married already?" behind which is the more important question for each individual to answer for himself, "How well do I know myself?" Admittedly then, there are absurd expectations and crippling demands imposed upon single persons in our society, including the divorced and the widowed. This unfortunate situation is easier to complain about than to remedy, for a very complex reason dealing with our misunderstanding of the nature of shame and guilt. It is easy to blame antiquated and barbaric laws dealing with sex behavior, but the laws themselves are a reflection of mainstream American morality which can be reshaped and reformulated only if enough responsible people speak out and only if enough people with integrity break through conventionalism and let their behavior shine as a saner way. This takes the courage of those who can remain unshameable.

CHAPTER 3

Love and Love and Love

T HERE IS NO REALITY AS DIFFI-
cult to grasp conceptually as the experience of love. True, no
matter what we try to say about any essential dimension of
life, words are inadequate. We can only project the shadow
of our experiences in speech or writing or some art form. Yet,
since language is one of the primary modes of communication, use it we must.

The impoverishment of English words and phrases with
which to convey love-feelings and experiences is indicative of
a basic cultural problem—a problem which is perhaps universal
and existential, the dilemma of being human. For reasons
still not adequately understood, we find it difficult to be at
ease with, to accept comfortably and joyously, our own flesh
or body. It is deceptively easy to blame this problem on "Vic-
torianism," or "Puritanism," or "parental or societal repres-
sion," or "theological or philosophical dualism." Such concepts
do point toward important and partially true insights, but
ultimately they are academic descriptions which only beg the
question. It seems as if every age of man has been pressed
with this problem and forced to come to terms with it in
some way or other.

We in our time and society are ambivalent with respect to
the healthy incorporation of the body into the self-image. We
are obsessed with the beautification of the body. Vast commercial enterprises cater to and create anxiety about our concern for looking trim, smelling inoffensively, and looking
masculine or feminine. If we do not meet these commercial-

ized standards, the dire consequences are vividly impressed upon us by advertisements: We will be unloved and miss the enjoyment of a full life. It is not that these diets, deodorants, and directives for dynamic sensuality are bad or wrong in themselves. It is what they hide and miss that makes them so subtly threatening to our happiness. In our pursuit of acceptable appearance we tend to neglect the necessary attention to more significant aspects of our being. With some sophistication it is relatively easy to acquire marks of attractiveness and the characteristics of sex appeal. But what we feel or fail to feel inside is another story. Confidence in looking lovely does not guarantee confidence in feeling loveable.

One of the many reasons for this is that we feel estranged from our bodies. The outline may be alluring, the deodorant or perfumes exotic, the hairdo fashionable, and the clothes chic, but underneath the clothing there are those hidden parts with those unmentionable functions. The erotic becomes suppressed, if not repressed, and left to the privacy of fantasy and the pursuit of the "perverts," while "love" is sentimentalized as an affair of the heart and idealized as a communion of souls. Certainly, love involves the heart and the soul, but it also involves the body. Both the spirit and the flesh are willing, and together, not separately, they comprise the whole person.

Qualities of Love   The preceding remarks about the importance of the body are mentioned in order for our consideration of love to be grounded in the concreteness of our existence; whatever love may be, it involves matter as well as mind, sensuality as well as spirituality.

Love is not a simple emotion or relationship. There are qualities of interpersonal relationships which we characterize by a value judgment called loveable as opposed to hateful, affirmative rather than negative, enhancing rather than destructive. Perhaps, then, there are qualities of loving which correspond to differing qualitative relationships which, if analyzed, will bring us to a fuller understanding of what it means to love, both in terms of our own needs and the needs of the other. Using this approach, it seems to me that there are three basic types or dimensions of interpersonal relationships which elicit three qualities of love. We are attracted to others through lust for them; we relate to others because of friendship with them; and we become involved with people simply because they are living beings. Our single English word "love" confuses the meanings of these various relationships, and it will therefore be necessary to resort to hyphenated terms roughly analogous to the ancient Greek words for love: *eros, philia,* and *agape.* The corresponding three qualities of loving are: lust-love, friendship-love, and empathy-love. These loves are not mutually exclusive and can be felt at the same time by one person toward another. Furthermore, each of these love qualities has a spectrum of possibilities which continually shift, making for numerous and intriguing combinations. Therefore, the meaning of being in love differs not only from one person to another but changes continually within any given individual and also between any two persons.

Lust-love   Lust is a natural power of attraction which transforms us from mere insensate objects to responsive subjects; it is a magnetism deep in ourselves pulling us toward other people. Its range of feeling is very wide, encompassing the earthy and the esthetic. Modern views of man have tended to perpetuate the old theological or philosophical dualisms which relegate lust to biological or animalistic drives or instincts. I prefer, however, to understand lust as a human phenomenon, believing that all three love qualities are innate with wide ranges and varying intensities shaped by learning, experience, and individually given constitutional and psychological factors. We are caught in a very limited and impoverished conceptual framework when we think of love as pure, divine, selfless—in short, spiritual—while at the same time we degrade biological need, physical attraction, lust—in short, sensuality. The needs and impulses of the body are not "lower" or "baser" than the needs of the embodied self. What is lower or debasing, as opposed to higher or uplifting, is the manner in which any given individual combines and expresses the love qualities in any given situation. Lust, friendship, and compassion may be thought of as respectively earthy, earthly, and ethereal, but no one of these love qualities is superior to another; all three must be constructively integrated in the whole person. Regardless of what view each of us may hold concerning the origin and development of homo sapiens, we cause emotional blocks and confusion of values when we think of love as spiritual for civilized man in contrast to love as sex for primitive man. It seems more reasonable to assume that mankind has always been endowed with the ability to feel simultaneously these three love qualities. Our difficulty is that we do not know best how to handle this richness of our nature.

Lust-love is an energizer of our being. It moves us to seek out others of the opposite sex, to receive from them the fulfillment of our manifold needs, and to lavish upon them values which we need to actualize. It is an exhilarating dimension of life, the impulse behind man-woman game playing. The language of lust-love can be coarse as in off-color jokes, quaintly circumspect as in blushing love letters, or sensitively and beautifully erotic as in romantic poetry. There are but few primary experiences as stimulating and pleasurable as the imagination's embrace of a lovely person. This is an instinctive response to beauty perceived everywhere in the magnificence of nature's phenomena. Admittedly, "sex appeal" has different meanings to each man and woman. Yet, though its definition may be elusive, each individual knows when he feels attraction, deep attraction, lust-love, for someone of the opposite sex. Men seem to be more obvious in their relish of an exquisite woman and sometimes ogle in a rude manner, the workings of their imagination being quite transparent. But women not only accept and appreciate the role of being looked at and desired; they, too, allow their imagination to work. Flirtation is the name of the game inspired by lust-love. In the tender throes of courtship lovers may vow "I'll only have eyes for you," but it is not long after marriage before those eyes may take in a lot more than the beloved. While many people equate flirtation with temptation, such an activity can be a healthy and happy manifestation of lust-love both before and after marriage. The potential interpersonal dangers of flirting lie not in the activity itself, but in the foolish interpretation of it by insecure and possessive partners who see it as a threat to themselves. Because we try to sweep lust-love under the band of the engagement or wedding ring and deny it a function in our normal lives, we allow its power to become demonic rather than wholesome. There is much more to lust-love than the achievement of orgasm. There is also the delight in simply contemplating the loveliness of another, of innocently touching another, of hearing the voice or feeling the warm presence of another. We make a mistake in habitually attributing sinister or devious motives to one who seeks only a smile or a cordial greeting. It may seem naïve to attribute such simple satisfactions to the flirtations of the vast majority of people and, admittedly, there is always a risk in such open interest in and expression of lust. This is the case especially in a society which has so many immature if not harmful sexual misconceptions, restrictions, and practices. Yet it is precisely because our literature is so full of condemnations of lust and our upbringing so traditionally distrustful of sensuality that the positive aspects of this quality of love need to be strongly emphasized. Lust-love involves sex that is genital, biological, and procreational, and it also involves sexuality which is nongenital and makes life so much worth living.

This nongenital aspect of lust-love is very hard for many people to understand since our stereotypes of masculinity and femininity and making love are so shallow. We are led in popular literature to believe that the man strives mightily for the quick, big, awesome erection, and that woman strives for and is satisfied mightily by the explosive, shattering, and mystical orgasm. Certainly men and women do delight in their respective experiences of erection and penetration and mutual orgasm. Yet, it should also be realized that while lust-love may involve such experiences, it often involves something else: the sheer sensuality and intimacy of *being-with*. Modern men and women are cursed with the myth of the ultimacy of the orgasm. We are besieged with manuals which detail techniques for the achievement of sex climax, and we have sadly allowed ourselves to be defined as performing sexual beings in terms of narrow and rigid physiological satisfaction. While the delight of a satisfying mutual orgasm cannot be denied, we may lose sight of the more embracing reality of two persons revealing themselves one to another in nakedness and trust and tenderness. It is worthy of note that the ancient biblical description of carnal intimacy was rooted in the concept "to know." "To know" another sexually means much more than to feel the height or climax of physiological stimulation; it means as well, and perhaps more importantly, to be close to, to be with, to feel with, to understand the other.

Friendship-love   Lust-love, awakening us to the earthy and esthetic delights of sensuality, can also lead us into interpersonal or psychological trouble when it is indiscriminate, undisciplined, and selfish. A narrow and unrefined kind of lust leads to promiscuity, the abuse of relationships to satisfy the whim of the moment without consideration of the other. Promiscuity lacks the sense of *being-with*. It takes the ingredient of friendship-love mingled with lust-love to keep lust-love from degenerating into thoughtless, egocentric pleasure seeking.

Friendship-love includes a relational range from familiarity to intimacy. There are always a few acquaintances whom we want to know more closely. We feel comfortable with them, enjoy their presence, and share significant experiences with them. Friendship is not easy to achieve. Ideally, it allows the social masks to be shed; it reveals the person with all of his weaknesses and failures along with his admirable qualities. It does not abrogate evaluation and criticism, rather it transcends it, enabling an appreciation of the total person in encounter with another. Such solid, mutual relational affection is rare because we most often strive so consciously to project a loveable image. In doing so we are inclined to show others only a superficially better self and withdraw from self-exposure which might reveal too much of us to the perceptive other. All of us need at least a few persons in our lives with whom the interpersonal game playing is at a minimum. Otherwise we are always role playing and can get so adaptable in this that we can become confused as to who we really are. To be familiar with another obviates the censoring of every personal thought and feeling. It is a relationship which allows the sharing of private meanings, meanings of involvement which a third person would not fully understand because he is not part of an experience-between-two.

Friendship-love may not involve physical intimacy, especially when this relationship is between two persons of the same sex. It is interesting to note, however, that even when this is the case there are embraces, warm handclasps, or shoulder slaps. In the case of friends of opposite sexes, there may be greater degrees of physical intimacy, especially if mutual lust-love is also felt. Such intimacy may range from kissing to coitus, depending upon the mutual needs, circumstances, and understandings of the persons involved.

A phenomenal aspect of friendship-love is that it can contribute strength and sanity to a person's life even when the friend in question has not been seen for many years, or even if the friend has died. The memory of friendship is ineradicable, and there is a sense in which friends we have known become incorporated into our existence for life.

Empathy-love   If we summarize lust-love as *appreciation-of* and friendship-love as *being-with*, we can focus on the essence of empathy-love as *identity-with*. Just as friendship-love personalizes lust-love, empathy-love universalizes friendship-love. If we are privileged to know humanness through friendship, we are better able to realize emotionally, not merely intellectually, our oneness with the Family of Man. The suffering of all men is the suffering of each man; the tragedy of all, the tragedy of each; the glory of all, the glory of each. Empathy-love enables us to see each man as Everyman. All of us bleed, cry, laugh, despair, and hope alike, and that which distinguishes us culturally or racially ought to be seen as enriching rather than divisive. The relational range of empathy-love is from pity to compassion. At the very least, we should have the capacity to encounter those we consider to be less fortunate in life's circumstances with a sense of humility and wonder. "There, but for the grace of God, go I," is the traditional sentiment which points toward this mystery that I am I, born in this time and place and under these circumstances *instead of*. In its more active form, empathy involves us in the destiny of humanity through compassion. We love others simply because they, like we, are human and share identical challenges to survival and happiness. National, cultural, and ethnic content may differ, but underneath all is the same. It is the genius of the heroes of all religions that they were able to convey a concern and a message for the wholeness of all men: humanity. Empathy-love keeps friendship-love from idolatry and parochialism, from delusions between two. It provides us with a vision, a value system out of which evaluation of friendships is healthy and positive. It keeps us from remaining frozen in a narrow life of personal security and calls forth from us the wisdom and courage which is willing to risk even friendship for universal causes. Empathy-love is freely given. There is no calculated self-benefit or reward. We care simply because the other is, and that which is deepest in us is in all. Empathy-love is paradoxical in that it is a concern for all persons without the necessity of experience with all peoples. We can love Russians and Buddhists without knowing a Russian or a Buddhist.

A Model of Love   The ideal of love is a misleading preoccupation. What we commonly think of as love is instead a *process* of interaction among these three qualities of loving. We understand something about lust, friendship, and empathy, yet we have missed the value of each of these qualities of loving while we have pursued some ideal condition of love separate from these love qualities. We have been on the wrong track searching for a Platonic essence which has no relevance to existence. Instead of asking ourselves, "Am I in love?" we ought to ask, "What kinds of loving do I feel toward this person?" When we ask the first question, there can be no reasonable analysis of our needs and feelings which will allow us to make appropriate responses to the combination of love qualities we feel. But by asking ourselves the second question—assuming that we can give ourselves honest answers—we have more reasonable guidelines to shape our response to any loving encounter with another person. For example, the framework of three love qualities is helpful in the understanding of parent-child in-loveness. When a parent and a child of the opposite sex have a relationship qualitatively different from a parent and a child of the same sex, everybody concerned somehow feels apprehensive. The obvious is missed. For, according to the love-quality perspective, a mother will inevitably feel a different loving combination to a son than to a daughter because lust-love is a predictable interaction between different sexes. Also, the need to feel motherly or fatherly is not necessarily a psychological sub-limation because we can feel strong empathy-love toward a marriage partner without having to conclude that our "love" is immature. Mother-love is vastly exaggerated. Fathers can have the same empathy-love for their children as can mothers. Parental love is basically empathy with a hope for friendship and with a controlled minimum of lust. Too, a child will, because of his sex, have different love combinations toward the mother and the father and ought not to feel guilty about a given sexuality. These relational feelings are natural and are not "complexes." Such a term should be reserved only for clear-cut cases of a short circuit in the growing up relational process.

We come, then, to the admission that "love" is a compli-cated process involving at least three differentiated qualities of loving. When we "love" a particular person we are feeling some interaction of lust, friendship, and empathy, and our responsibility is to admit to ourselves which of these qualities is predominant and to shape our actions accordingly.

One final reflection. All three of these love qualities are good—human—in and of themselves, and no matter where we start, if we have patience and trust, we will, in all proba-bility, know the other two love experiences in our lifetime.

CHAPTER 4

Self-Enjoyment

MASTURBATION IS ONE OF THE
basic pleasures we enjoy from childhood through senility. In
every phase of our maturation this act of self-enjoyment as-
sumes different meanings yet almost always contributes to our
well-being. It should be unnecessary in this day and age to
make more than a casual passing reference to masturbation,
for its inevitability and benefits should be taken as much for
granted as the act of breathing. It is only when we suffer from
lack of air that breathing becomes a problem; it is only when
we cannot feel pleasure from the stimulation of our own
genitals that masturbation becomes a problem. Obviously,
compulsive masturbation may be symptomatic of emotional
difficulties as is, for example, compulsive overeating. But
masturbation in and of itself is not the cause of problems and
in most cases helps to keep emotional stresses within manage-
able bounds. This form of sensuality is neither a moral, medical, or psychological disorder except when ignorance or archaic
prejudices cause misconceptions and unhealthy attitudes which
in turn create problems. It is not worth the time to repeat
here the old wives' tales and the religious and medical fables
which sought to frighten youth with the supposed horrors
and evils of masturbation. We should relegate such stories to
the limbo of historical curiosity (sympathizing with the attempts of past generations to cope with the mysteries of
man's sexual nature) and concentrate on the positive aspects
of this form of self-enjoyment.

Accepting Yourself   From the moment we are born—

31

and perhaps even in the womb—we begin to explore, experiment with, and refine responses to our given sensuality. We are, after all, blessed with an abundance of sensual capacities and needs which are eventually channeled into modes of social propriety, and in the process the richness of our corporeal being suffers partial stultification. That which serves the total social good as it is understood in any given cultural period takes precedence over individual self-realization. Happily, individuals usually have more sense than societies, and it is the tension between prophets and masses which sets the conditions for progress. The progress of civilization can be gauged by the degree of social consensus and individual freedom operative at any given time. One of the tasks of today's younger generation is to maximize sexual freedom while, at the same time, maintaining essential, cohesive, time-proven social values. Obviously, within this wider framework of social concern masturbation can hardly be considered a threat to civilization. On the contrary, because it is a means of self-discovery and self-acceptance it gives us greater self-knowledge and greater self-confidence, enabling us to be stronger participants in the shaping of the social order.

Self-knowledge is more than an exercise of the mind. It is also a matter of familiarity with one's own body and an exercise of all the functions of that body. It is critically important for our total health that we be comfortable with our being and that we know and use not only our nonphysical capacities but also our muscles, physical senses, and sex organs. Our genitals are, after all, a part of us, and we should realize that their function is not only procreative but erotic and pleasurable as well. It is ridiculous to assume that these parts of the self must lie in state until the awakening of the honeymoon. On the contrary, who would propose that the best way to train a marathon runner would be to keep him in a wheelchair from birth in order to save his legs for the big race? It is healthful that we should experiment with self-stimulated orgasm and incorporate this experience and self-familiarity into our total self-image before we attempt to respond as total, integrated persons with another.

Helping Your Lover to Love You To "make love" is to learn pleasure giving. This art is discussed more fully in the following section on mutual masturbation but requires brief mention here. How are you to help your love partner to have the pleasure of satisfying you if you are afraid to touch yourself and discover your own pattern of excitation and orgasm? This question applies to both men and women. If you know the delight of touching yourself you will be more empathetic and responsive to the need of your love partner to be lovingly caressed, thus making coitus not just a transaction of rights and duties but a rich exchange of endearment. An interesting present-day phenomenon is the apparent increase in homosexuality in men over sixty, even among those who are married. One of the probable reasons for this is the lack of patience and consideration on the part of wives who do not give enough time and stimulation to the art of touching. Most likely, however, these same men have not devoted enough care to this identical need on the part of their wives, with the sad result that both spouses have missed the full dimension of tenderness throughout their married years. Right attitudes toward the values of masturbation while people are young and single can help them bring more of themselves to their marriages and enable them to contribute more to the satisfaction of their partners even throughout old age.

Your Private World of Fantasy Masturbation is a relaxation of both physical and psychic tension. Children engage in the activity simply because it feels good, sometimes doing it while daydreaming, watching television, or reading a book. It is an innocent pastime of "playing with oneself." By the onset of puberty the fantasies associated with masturbation assume explicit sexual content, content which becomes more vigorously and imaginatively lustful through the progress of adolescence. The fantasy content and meanings of the act change after marriage. Married people may occasionally masturbate for various positive reasons, and in old age, especially in widowhood, it is a time not only for relaxing tension but for precious memories.

Masturbation is a private act with personal meanings. It is a unique experience which has validity in and of itself. In healthy adolescents filled with eager yearning and strong desire, it can serve as a pressure valve to powerful emotions. The accompanying fantasies should not be considered "dirty thoughts" but the natural imaginations of lust which everyone except the emotionally disturbed can contain and express at appropriate times in moral circumstances. Lustful thinking, no matter how bizarre, is not immoral. These moments of private physical and psychic self-discovery are necessary for inner equilibrium and mental health.

CHAPTER 5

The Pleasures of Petting

THE FULL RANGE OF INTERPER-
sonal enjoyment comes into play when one progresses from
necking, or passionate kissing, to petting, an encounter which
involves feeling and stimulating the partner's genitals and
erotic zones. Petting is intensely pleasurable and exciting—
pleasurable because areas of the body are aroused to greater
sensitivity, and exciting because such activity is qualitatively
different from previous experiences. At best, it is a precious
experience remembered for a lifetime. For many, however,
the first involvement in petting is remembered as an anxious
and embarrassing, if not guilt-producing, experience.

The reasons for the negative feelings are many, the most
obvious of which is the assumption that such intimacy before
marriage is morally wrong. Parents, religious instructors, teachers, and other societal authorities have taught us that such
activity is wrong. But these authorities are irresponsible in
that they rarely explicitly or rationally *teach* us why they believe petting to be wrong; they merely imply or hint their dis-
approval with forbidding and forboding warnings. Girls are
warned to be "nice," boys are told not to be "fresh." They
are told not to be "impure," "promiscuous," "lascivious,"
"dirty," etc., etc. Parents, of course, with rare exception, never
talk about the subject openly. Parents tend to have a head-in-
the-sand morality which fosters noncommunication with their
children. And this, as far as youth is concerned is probably
just as well. For the parental conspiracy of silence leaves
young adults some room to be comfortable with their own

feelings and experiments. As long as girls keep from becoming pregnant, and as long as boys keep from "getting girls into trouble," this sexual middle-ground of petting is presumed to be nonexistent. Indeed, it is ironic that parents feel reassured about their children's "normalcy" if they are popular and have many dates; parents don't seem to be conscious of the pressures for petting. Insofar as children *are* taught sophisticated reasons for not petting, they probably hear one of three arguments: a) petting inevitably leads to intercourse; b) petting is a form of exploitation or use of the other person; c) petting leads only to psychological and physical frustration, thereby causing maladjustment in marriage. For the moment, we shall ignore the "reason" petting is "wrong," for this is no reason at all, but simply a value judgment which presumes reasons. Let us consider these three arguments against petting.

Petting as a Path to Coitus

There are reasonable precautions against petting which are based on the assumption that two persons who pet are headed for coitus. It is a fact that some couples who excite each other sexually, especially if they have comfortable privacy for any length of time, will engage in coitus. This often happens when the boy gets aggressive and the girl doesn't know how to stop him. Or it happens when the couple gets carried away and, because they have to prove something about their manliness or womanliness, go "all the way." Such cases, however, do not prove that coitus with a specific petting partner is inevitable or unavoidable. Rather, insofar as negative motives are involved coitus occurs because of erroneous ideas about what it is to be a man or a woman. Because of personality or character weaknesses some young men and women will be headed for premarital and marital difficulties in spite of what is taught to them.

Those who assume that petting inevitably leads to coitus fail to recognize the subtle meanings of intimacy for those who are engaged to be married or who are married, as compared to those who are unattached and still discovering sexuality. Engaged couples who are very serious about marriage after a while see no sense in stopping at petting, for it is, for them, an arbitrary stopping point. They are deeply committed to each other and, by using contraceptives, feel free to enjoy each other physically. Indeed, far too many are much too casual about intercourse without contraceptives, either assuming foolishly that contraceptives are vulgar or impediments to pleasure, or merely feeling that pregnancy before the formal exchange of marriage vows is a relatively minor matter. Our contemporary cultural sex standards are quite liberal and lenient toward those who are engaged.

For those who are married petting is, obviously, an entirely different experience. Petting is considered "foreplay," designed to warm the partners to the final consummation in coitus. More will be said about foreplay in subsequent sections. Let it suffice to say now that petting for unattached young adults is not foreplay. *It is a valuable end in itself*. This assertion will be elaborated upon in the remainder of this chapter.

Petting as Exploitation of Persons

The charge of exploitation or the use of persons is most often leveled against those who engage in premarital coitus. It is also used as an argument against petting and must be considered.

Again, there is sound advice in this precaution. When authorities—parental, religious, educational, or societal—tell us, "No," or "Don't," it is not out of some diabolical desire to make us unhappy or chained to the past. Rules and prohibitions are founded on the reflective experience of individuals or groups who seek to uphold certain higher values, and to spare us as much pain and anguish as possible. Rules and prohibitions must, however, be examined and re-evaluated in each generation. In this case, the precaution against using people can teach us important guiding principles for interpersonal relationships. Take the double standard as an example. Boys exploit girls out of their own insecurity concerning their masculine self-image. The "conquest" is primary and the girl insignificant. Fortunately, this manner of behavior is becoming archaic as the sexual revolution progresses and the war between the sexes ceases. Increasingly, as an ethic of regard for the female as a person is forged, the braggart who boasts a "feel" or a "lay" is looked upon with disfavor. Nevertheless, ego-building sexual experiences of the male are often at the expense of the female who is treated as a thing of momentary pleasure. Girls, on the other hand, have their own motivations and techniques for using boys as rungs on the popularity ladder. Most often there is no conscious attempt to use or hurt, but the need to prove something to oneself is so overwhelming that the feelings of, and consequences to, the partner are secondary, if considered at all. There certainly are, then, ways in which men and women use each other—or to be more to the point, *abuse* each other. The interpersonal abuses of some, however, should not be allowed to define the intimacy standards of all. For there is a profound sense of goodness and beauty in two persons who use each other for the fulfillment of mutual needs and desires. The world of the adolescent and young adult can be a lonely world. The experience of closeness, tenderness, and discovery which petting provides is one of the most precious and sacred experiences of life. Two people expose themselves to each other, and a new world of joyfulness unfolds. It really does not matter what the precise motivation is of each; all that matters is that two people open themselves to one another in trust and with feelings of wonder and exhilaration. This contact for them is infinitely more significant than sensual contact, as beautiful as that is. It unlocks new dimensions of self, of relatedness, of reality. Yet, everyone needs to be held and caressed, to be treasured, and to feel sensually alive. It is in this sense that petting is an end in itself and has meanings and an impact qualitatively different from the relationships of engagement and marriage. Indeed, most young adults are not primarily seeking coitus. Rather, they are seeking a warm and loving relationship within which coitus is incidental and even unnecessary. Free yourself from the erroneous presumption that you have to go beyond petting to be a "real" man or woman. Furthermore, realize that there is no cause for shame in petting or for an everlasting commitment to those with whom you are privileged to share unique and intimate relationships. It is enough that for a time two persons reached out and blessed one another with the concreteness of their being.

The "why" of petting is not as practical a consideration as the "with whom." They are, of course, interrelated, but the practical question is very important and more subject to understanding and control. Petting for reasons of higher popularity ratings, for example, is a self-defeating enterprise because neither the means nor the end is ultimately satisfactory. Sex as a proving ground is no proving ground at all, but merely a game of self-deception with consequences which range from frustration to tragedy. Indulgence in petting is, of course, not tragic in itself, regardless of motivation or partner. Far more serious, for example, is the risk of riding in a car with an idiot who has to show off and ends up demolishing the car and maiming or killing you. The proper assessment of the personality and character of a date in the matter of responsible driving habits is, literally, a matter of life and death. Petting is relatively harmless by contrast, for the psychic wounds which result from an interpersonal collision are mild—relative to death. But relative to life, psychic scars are a deeply serious matter. Whom you seek for a relationship of closeness says as much about you as about the other person. The kind of person with whom you are intimate reflects your image of yourself and subsequently shapes your attitudes and opinions toward many important matters for the rest of your life. What is being said, then, is that each person should not abuse others or allow their own self or integrity to be abused in the ignorant assumption that this is an inconsequential matter. You ought to be highly selective in your petting experiences, being deliberate in your assent at certain times with certain people, and very firm in your refusal with certain other people. Know your partner well, and if you respect him or her, enjoy his or her company, and know him well enough to *talk* about limits and expectations, then you need not be afraid that the experience will be negative for either. Obviously, one can never guarantee or have complete foreknowledge of the meaning or impact of a given experience upon someone else; it is enough to know that your decision was thoughtful and responsible. The mutual physical use of two persons—a use which is not only sensually pleasant but psychologically positive—is a worthwhile risk in the struggle to mature and to know who you are.

Petting as Physically Frustrating

It is possible that many instances of premarital petting result in physical frustration for the man, rather than for both. The petting is often brief and occurs in the most unusual places and situations that allow little privacy. Furthermore, if you have not talked about intimacy with your partner, there may be conflicts in expectation which cause hurt and misunderstanding. Even if time, place, and person all seem reasonably right, one or the other may bring some unrealistic or pseudoscientific notions to the situation. One such questionable notion is that coitus is the only normal result of petting. People accept this idea because they think either that stopping short of orgasm is harmful or that a normal man or woman should go all the way. Nonsense! Petting without orgasm or coitus—for persons with a mature relationship and attitude—is not harmful nor does it indicate any inadequacy, physical or emotional.

Young adults, in high school, or later, who indulge in petting without disciplined examination of self and situation are foolish, and are likely to be carried toward disastrous coital experiences which leave either psychic scars or result in pregnancy. Others, however, may be ready for petting and to go even further in satisfying each other to the point of mutual orgasm *without coitus*. This activity involves mutual masturbation which, as difficult as it is to discuss, needs to be openly considered.

The Benefits of Mutual Masturbation

Mutual masturbation is a taboo topic. It is acceptable when considered in marriage manuals under the category of foreplay but few parents allow themselves to think that their children could ever contemplate this pleasure, let alone indulge in it. But mutual masturbation between young adults has several benefits which most parents should admit. Again, it is important to realize that parents are not suppressive because of an arbitrary impulse to deny pleasure or rewarding experiences. Rather, it is a complex case of a generation gap—a gap which, in our times, spans a major evolutionary step in sex ethics.

Before four benefits of mutual masturbation are discussed, let us remember that these benefits are of the greatest value only to those who are ready to accept the experience without guilt, to those who have a partner with similar values, and to those who have the opportunity for such activity in a place which allows for adequate time, privacy, and relaxation. The four benefits are not the only possible ones and are not discussed in an order of priority. In talking about mutual masturbation we are, of course, referring to an act in which two persons stimulate each other to the point of orgasm.

Release of Sex Tension   It might seem that consideration of sexual tension contradicts previous assertions that petting can be an end in itself. If one pets, isn't it important or necessary to have release in orgasm? Such is not necessarily the case. Sometimes, after a petting session, one or both partners may masturbate at a later time in the privacy of his or her bedroom. But it should be realized that sexual tensions exist most of the time. The feelings of lust aroused by the sight of a beautiful person of the opposite sex, movies, television, reading materials, or mere thought can also result in masturbation. Sexual tension is a normal condition of life, and most of the time we are unaware of it. There are also unconscious ways in which we achieve psychic and physical equilibrium: dreams, fantasy, creative activity, and physical exertion. But, if we are ready for the experience of mutual masturbation and would like to seek its enjoyment as a direct means of acting out sexual tension, this activity can be most satisfying.

Exposure of Self   Mutual masturbation is more than masturbation. It involves contact with another person and requires an exposure of ourself which masturbation in isolation cannot provide. Masturbation, mutual masturbation, and coitus are qualitatively different orders or levels of sexuality which are all worthwhile in themselves and are never merely substitutes for one or the other. This exposure is obviously physical, but it is also existential and psychological. Once having participated in it you will never be the same person you were. Your image of yourself will change, your feelings toward and opinions about your friend will change, and your insights and understandings of the opposite sex will change. Hopefully, all such changes will be enriching and rewarding.

Being naked in the presence of a lover is a revealing situation. It reveals your body, obviously. But the reactions of the other toward your naked body, as you perceive them consciously and unconsciously, will reveal to you something about yourself and the nature of the opposite sex. You, with all of your anxieties and self-doubts, will have a new feeling toward yourself if, when in the presence of another in full nakedness, you are accepted and treated with tenderness and respect. You will find it an exhilarating and happy experience which can enable you to shed all fears of sexuality and all doubts about your possibly being an undesirable person. Human flesh will lose its potential fearfulness and, in sensing yourself valued, enjoyable, and pleasure-giving, you will walk and live with a new sense of ease and confidence. Constantly assaulted by the communications media with unrealistic sexual messages and pictures, you will find a sense of comfortableness with yourself, even though you are not a perfect specimen of Mr. or Miss America. One can be far from an "ideal" physical specimen and still be desired and enjoyed. As you are accepted, so you will be better able to accept yourself and others.

Familiarity and Communication   Learning about sexual expectations, desires, and responses of the opposite sex is no small accomplishment. Such lessons can be learned to your benefit before marriage or before you are driven into an early marriage because of your sexual needs. It is a tragedy of our contemporary culture that sexual experience and marriage are thought to be irrevocably united. It is not that sex before marriage guarantees or even makes easier the success of a particular marriage. Rather, it is a probability that marriage can be more worthwhile and creative if it is based on important factors other than the need and desire for sex. Premarital sex can help you become familiar with methods of giving as well as receiving pleasure. The responsibilities of the male for sexually satisfying the female to the point of orgasm have been explicitly detailed for several decades. What is equally important, though discussed less frequently, is the responsibility of the female to learn and apply methods for allowing the male maximum sexual enjoyment and pleasure. It is taken for granted that boys derive pleasure from stimulating the breasts and vulva of the girl, both manually and orally. We should assume that girls also can enjoy the manual and oral stimulation of the penis. The extent to which they cannot do so is due to the girl's *and boy's* sad misconception that such acts are not proper for "good" girls and that they are only performed by prostitutes. If prostitutes have any secret about satisfying men, it is their observation from experience that there is no magic in the penis. For this organ does not sping erect merely because the male thinks about sex or is in bed with a naked woman. Women, too, ought to learn the techniques and the patience which help the man to relax and become stimulated to the point of erection. This ability is especially important in later years when the man requires as much tender preparation for orgasm as does the woman. A girl who learns to enjoy masturbating her boyfriend will hopefully rid herself of nonsensical notions of "virility" which plague both men and women. In any case, though specific advice from marriage counselors and sexologists will change from time to time as greater knowledge of physiological and psychosexual responses is gained, every man and woman can learn a great deal about mutual pleasure giving and receiving by using common sense in healthful intimate relationships. There is variation in female orgasm patterns and also in the kinds and length of stimulation required for male erection. No given individual will match precisely the descriptions and graphs in manuals and textbooks. Indeed, no written work can ever capture fully the dynamics of sexual exchange felt by each individual. Thus, mutual masturbation can be helpful in becoming familiar with the responses of a particular person, can give insight into one's own preferences and responses, and can provide helpful guidelines for future intimate encounters. Also, the experience may teach us that "sex" is not a grim or awesome sacrosanct encounter. There is humor and lightness of heart in the naked frolic which makes us glad to be alive and appreciative of the fullness of our sensual nature.

What is done and not done during these moments of physical excitement can help you also to understand dimensions of nonverbal physical communication. Too, what is said and not said can bring you to a fuller awareness of what another person is like when he is confronted on a far deeper level of relationship than usual social roles permit. Such knowledge is perhaps too wonderful and too high for us to assimilate fully, but it can increase our sensitivity in human relationships to such a degree that life can be richer than it might otherwise have been. It is also possible that in having satisfactory orgasm with a thoughtfully selected partner, the person will be left in fuller control of his sexual needs and desires and freer in the many other pursuits and interests of life. With tensions decreased, with greater joyfulness of being, with increased awareness of the uniqueness of others, one is apt to be a more complete human being worth more to himself and, consequently, worth more to society and mankind.

Uses in Marriage   To know the refinements and nuances of manual and oral sexual stimulation is to bring more to marital sex. This does not mean, however, that this art cannot be happily and satisfactorily learned after marriage. Indeed, those who decide that premarital sex is immoral will have their most complete sexual fulfillment only within marriage. However, those who can conscientiously enjoy premarital sex in situations they consider moral, can bring to their marriages attitudes and experiences allowing for anxiety-free, intense, and varied marital sex. Mutual masturbation in marriage is usually considered second-best to coital orgasm, a method to be used as an expedient when "normal" orgasm cannot, for some reason, be achieved. All of the manual and oral techniques of mutual masturbation are considered as preliminary warm up or foreplay to the great climax of coitus. What must be frankly stated is that mutual masturbation to the point of orgasm can be a complete and enjoyable sexual act even in marriage. Much too much has been made of the ecstasy of simultaneous orgasm in coitus. There are even those who maintain that the male ejaculation within the vagina is the only normal sexual act. But such opinions do not coincide with the experiences of many married couples. Like any aspect of the marriage relationship, the sexual act, performed in the traditional manner of coitus, can become quite routine and boring. Variety in stimulation and climax is necessary, and often the performance of mutual masturbation to orgasm is refreshing, welcome, and more satisfactory. Indeed, the artful use of hand, lips, tongue, and mouth can provide more intense and pleasurable orgasm than conventional coitus. It is also probable that most couples achieve orgasm not simultaneously but sequentially. This often means that the orgasm for the wife or husband is brought about in a masturbatory manner. Then there are times when both are not in the mood but one willingly masturbates the other, a loving gesture which gives pleasure to both.

These aspects of marital sex are mentioned to bring to our awareness some of the realities which may be encountered in marriage, and to suggest that the practice of mutual masturbation may provide partners with attitudes conducive to lustier and more delightful marital sex.

It is sad to realize that there are many marriages in which the partners have desires that they are afraid to express or ashamed to practice. Reading the terms "fellatio" and "cunnilingus" in antiseptic manuals or the vulgar synonyms which fill cheap novels doesn't help eradicate the unfortunate feelings that such sensual satisfaction is somehow perverse. Our language does not provide us with suitable phrases or words to express poetically or simply the joys of vigorous and complete sensual exploration. Someday, the vocabulary of intimacy will reflect more genuinely the beauty of true lovemaking. When our stated moral values catch up with our hidden practices, then, undoubtedly, we will permit our language to express aspects of sexual acts which we have had the good sense to enjoy all along. In the meantime, there are no embarrassments between people who are "simpatico," and there is fun and even sweet innocence in each couple creating their own syllabus of sex and lexicon of love.

CHAPTER 6

Going All the Way

Ⓘ T HAS PREVIOUSLY BEEN AS-
serted that petting and mutual masturbation can be enjoyable
activities in themselves and that such excitement does not
inevitably result in coitus. It must, however, be anticipated
that the person who has experienced pleasure in sexual intimacies will eventually feel ready to "go all the way," either
with the partner with whom he is comfortably familiar or
with a new partner who is also ready for, or who may already
have had, this satisfaction. It is to be hoped—and this should
be our goal—that it will happen in circumstances and in a
manner which enriches humanness, even though there will
forever remain an element of interpersonal risk in this act.
To expend energy and influence in exhorting young adults
never to engage in coitus before marriage is a quixotic enterprise which is ultimately a disservice to youth. Someday, family discussions about ground rules for sexual intimacy will be
as much taken for granted as casual instruction about such
commonplace matters as cleanliness, manners, and school-
work. One of the indispensable conditions for healthy participation in coitus is the use of reliable contraceptives. This
topic will be discussed in a following section. Our interest in
this chapter will be with the motivations, values, and hazards
of an encounter as old as mankind yet ever new, universal but
always unique, mysterious but quite revealing.

The Giving of Sex   Sex connection or coupling of organs is natural to human physiology and allows a vigor of
bodily expression and fulfillment which is valued equally by

men and women. There is nothing inherently passive about
the role of the woman in coitus. The pelvic response of thrust
is a natural bodily translation of psychic need which is gratify-
ing to both men and women; it is a movement resulting in a
feeling of completion when met by the factuality of the other.
The supposition that men are aggressive and women passive
must finally be laid to rest in the museum of folklore—a
quaint tale reflecting an exclusively male frame of reference.
It may give men of stone-age mentality ego satisfaction to
presume that they are sexually dominant and superior, but
this is an illusion which, if maintained, will cause only frustration and misunderstanding.

Sex is. It takes its rightful place with other natural functions of the human body and cannot be denied, yet society
still severely restricts its exercise. However, if men and women
will risk death testing themselves against mountains simply
because mountains are there, it is not surprising that they will
take the risks of coitus simply because the sex organs are
there. If there is any truth to the age-old gripe that the
natural state of the sexes is war, it is a truth applicable to
relational and psychological tensions and hostilities, not to
physiological compatibility. Man fits into woman; man comes
out of woman and suckles at her breasts; man and woman
need each other's bodies to be and to become fully alive. The
homosexual relationship does present a dramatic variation of
the compelling man-woman attraction. Since homosexuality
is considered elsewhere in this book, suffice it to say now that
even this human encounter is unusual precisely because of
the overpowering need for two persons of the same sex to relate through and enjoy each other's bodies. The communication and self-expression in the sexual act cannot be devalued
without distorting the personality to the great peril of both
individual sanity and societal health.

In the coital embrace, a man and a woman can experience

uniquely the beingness of sexuality; it is a mutual gift of self-knowledge with the potential for several other precious human exchanges. It can give comfort, pleasure, acceptance, and relief from emotional isolation as well as the relaxation of physical tension. If the solace, enjoyment, and self-realization of men and women experienced in coitus is wrong then something is wrong with reality.

Sex in Its Place   With a minimum of sexual arousal a woman can be accommodating—in this sense, passive—and cooperate with her partner for his pleasure. A man, however, when he is physically or emotionally exhausted, not in the mood, filled with too much alcohol, or even overexcited, cannot meet stereotyped expectations of lovemaking, that is, produce an immediate erection. Men, therefore, bear the burden of performance which leads to frustrations and disappointments on the part of both men and women who do not understand this fact. Such misunderstanding is truly sad, for the essence of lovemaking is not mutual orgasm but simply mutual intimacy. For this reason, satisfactory or unsatisfactory orgasm in premarital coitus is by no means a measure of the probable success or failure of a marriage. It is the quality of interpersonal relationship which matters, not the intensity of the orgasm. What is learned about sexuality is critically important, not how one performs sexually. For this reason, the trial and error of premarital coitus can be extremely valuable to a person's understanding of himself and of the opposite sex provided that the man and woman learn the art of intimacy without anxiety about orgasm. Everything that has previously been said about petting and mutual masturbation applies here. To be explicit about it: When the man finds that he does not have an erection merely because naked bodies are intertwined, and when the woman discovers that she is not glowing or has not achieved an orgasm merely upon being entered and receiving ejaculation, something profound has been realized by both! Simply explaining this reality to youth—the fact that there is no magic in coitus—is as fruitless as describing a sunset to a person unable to see color. It must be experienced. True, it is by no means necessary for this insight to be gained before marriage, but it can be helpful in that the limited values of coitus are realized and partners are chosen without sexual distortions and with proper focus upon the total issues and values involved in the marital commitment.

There are many values in life of greater worth than the one of pleasurable sex: To earn a child's respect as a parent; to be valued as a person by friends; to achieve a self-determined professional or vocational goal in spite of many obstacles; to be "turned on" to existence without the crutch of drugs or alcohol; to face with a "simpatico" marriage partner the lifelong challenge of leaving humanity the simple gift of life— a life which gave as well as received and left the world a better place for having been there. Viewed against these values, sex, in and of itself, is a commonplace and transitory enjoyment, as important as the delight of an ice cream cone to a child. And as ice cream devoured too quickly can cause a headache, coitus indulged in prematurely can create an emotional ache. Even married men and women may know this emotional ache in the form of a vague, unsettling depression which can be called the postcoital blues.

It happens something like this. A couple (they can, by the way, be of any age or marital status) is engaged in physical intimacy, relishing mutual stimulation, and absorbed in the exciting rise to climax. Suddenly, it is ended; both have had a satisfying orgasm and rest relaxed, the silence metered by heavy breathing. But the relaxation is only apparent. Actually, both are quietly avoiding any further encounter, for they are struck with the realization that they are lying next to a stranger and do not know what to do or say. They cannot even smile genuinely and say an honest "thank you" to each other—the exquisite ending of only experienced, unshameable persons. They are close—smells, tastes, and myriad physical impressions still linger—but they are locked inside their separateness and feel uncomfortable, if not threatened, by the exposure of themselves made to the other. Something is missing and this abrupt, empty experience is more than they had imagined. This is their emotional ache, their postcoital blues.

It can be helpful for this experience to be realized before marriage; it can be tragic after the vows have been exchanged. Why is it good as a premarital situation? Because the limitations of sex are discovered, and further growth and learning can take place, while the romanticized expectations of sex will not precipitate premature marriage. Young adults who have been wise enough to take contraceptive and interpersonal precautions to allow for a positive sex experience can absorb this commonplace aspect of sex emotionally and grow to the point of maturity where they can enjoy it for what it is and can have a warm, appreciative ending with their partner without disappointment or depression. This lesson can enable them to put sex in its most healthful perspective, to accept its limitations, to focus on a greater value context in choosing a partner for marriage, and ultimately to know that unspeakably joyous communion in a creative monogamous union.

In past generations, there have been valid reasons for an absolute prohibition against coitus before the wedding. That time is no more. On the contrary, it is the duty of the present generation of parents, and all who teach youth, to enable them to achieve a comfortable sexual intimacy, even to the degree of going all the way, which will help them in the contemporary long stretch of postadolescent singlehood as participating adults—young adults who, growing more secure within themselves and in their interpersonal relationships, to enrich the world of tomorrow.

Chastity, Virginity, and the Double Standard   Two letters, N and O, conjoined at the right time with moral fervor
can save a young man or woman painful regrets and destructive experiences. "No," however, is a long word, not easily
summoned, for it reaches deeply into character and personality. It can be a profound affirmation of self-respect. If we
have worked to develop essential character strengths, it will
be easier to master our involvements and refuse to participate
in acts we think improper. On the other hand, when prohibitions against certain acts are merely the commands of
external authorities which we obey because of possible pun-
ishment—authorities we have not accepted with understanding
—then we will drift, not really understanding why we
do what we do, and more often being a passive victim of
circumstances rather than a participant. It is assumed that it
is the girl who always bears the burden of saying "no," of
"drawing the line," but the enlightened boy who knows that
it is also his responsibility to resist the pressure to "make
out," also accepts the burden of decision. The death of the
double standard means not only that women are as free as
men to engage in premarital intimacy, it means that men are
as responsible as women for the quality of such relationships.
It is ironic that as sexual freedom increases in our culture, the
right to refuse intimacy with any particular person must be
firmly emphasized. Just because "everybody's doing it" and
"I don't want to be left without friends" are prevalent excuses, they are, nevertheless, excuses which indicate moral
weakness and lack of imagination in handling relationships.

When a young person confronts for the first time an
opportunity for premarital coitus, the response of "yes" or
"no" will probably depend on factors other than the traditional ideal of virginity; especially true for engaged couples
since an announcement of marriage is now widely accepted as
a license for sexual privileges. This engagement period is so-

ciety's compromise with premarital sex, and those who are willing to deceive themselves enough to play the game can have several engagements before marriage without suffering the reputation of being "promiscuous." For some persons in certain situations, however, the line just before "going all the way," may be reasonably drawn based on concerns for family, future spouse, self-respect, and psychological stability. The term virginity is used here in a basic sense: If a girl has received a penis in her vagina, she is no longer a virgin and neither is the boy who enters the girl. Thus, no matter what other forms of sexual intimacy a couple engages in, they are still virgins if they have never performed coitus.

For a person who lives in a small town or in a close neighborhood group, a sense of family honor can reinforce conservative sexual behavior. Parents can be deeply hurt and suddenly change their feelings and attitudes toward their own child if they discover from remarks made by neighbors that their "little girl" or "little boy" has been sexually "loose." There is a vast majority of young men and women who ask themselves as they face a questionable situation, "What would my mother and father think of me if they knew?" It is a pity that others don't bother to ask such a question because they know their parents don't care or because they never knew their parents well enough to feel their values and standards.

The double standard, unhappily, is still operative to some extent everywhere and especially within rural and certain ethnic segments of our country. It is still possible for a young woman to ruin her life by becoming involved with a man who brags about his "conquest," magnifying a harmless petting experience into an orgiastic episode. The girl then becomes typed as "one of those kind" and, out of bravado begins to try to act the role or, out of shame, withdraws in bitterness from social contacts. Thus, a wide range of possible future husbands is deprived her unless she leaves that environment for work or study in another setting where she can begin again. There are very good reasons for women to maintain virginity at least until engagement, and also to choose with care a partner for noncoital intimacy who is sensitive and discrete.

However, guilt can not easily be left behind and can create subtle but lasting effects in a relationship. If one believes, conscientiously, that coitus before engagement or marriage is morally wrong, yet gives in to please the partner in the hope of holding him, there will probably be negative attitudes linked with sex which will have to be worked out at some point in marriage. It is incredibly simple for couples to drift helplessly into a disastrous marriage by rationalizing the rightness of coitus with the assumption that they are engaged. Neither one is honest enough to admit that they merely wanted intimacy; getting engaged suddenly makes it right and they therefore do not have to confess doing something which they really feel was wrong. Many marriages are made of such delusions. At the foot of many an altar have stood white-veiled "virgins" bearing their babies. Premarital pregnancy need not, of course, weaken a marriage. But how much healthier it would be if those who believe in the importance of virginity hold to it without apology and, if they weaken, face their failure without using it as either blackmail or rationalization for marriage.

In support of the standard of virginity, there is wisdom in not taking the psychological risks of coitus. The postcoital blues have already been mentioned, and it must be recognized that the psychological makeup of some people causes severe depression after casual coital experience. Also, it is probable that the first attempts of most couples are humorous at best, if not dismally embarrassing. The young man either ejaculates too quickly or does not obtain erection, and his partner also feels inadequate because she doesn't know what to do and is usually left in a state of tension or befuddlement. It can be a very unpleasant experience with negative memories which distort future relationships. Love is never free; it involves a high price of involvement and a risky investment of psychic energy and moral commitment. Unless one has religious principles and a philosophy of sex which allow for the kind of guiltless and shame-free relaxed intimacy which has already been discussed, it is far better to hold the line of virginity and leave the risks of sexual experimenting to the more secure context of formal engagement or marriage.

The standard of virginity for both sexes is not irrelevant to contemporary man-woman relationships, and it can be a strong foundation for character and marriage for those wishing to live within this standard moral framework.

Chastity Without Virginity   "Chaste makes waste" is a slogan popular enough to have been made into a button but, though a catchy cliché, it is an irrelevant dictum. Chastity and virginity are separable issues. These terms have long been used as synonyms, and, indeed, they are closely connected in that "chaste" is used as a value judgment of virginity. In the future, however, dictionaries will not offer "virgin" as a primary meaning of "chaste," for increasingly among the younger generation it is recognized that a person may be one but not the other: chaste, but not a virgin; a virgin, but not chaste. One may, of course, be both or neither. Let us consider why it is valid for unmarried young adults who are nonvirgins conscientiously to consider themselves chaste.

Fortunately, there are many modern parents who are not worried about their children having premarital sexual experience. Rather, their concern is that their daughters and sons have responsible and healthy intimacies when and if they feel ready. The children of such parents do not, therefore, carry as great a burden of fear or anxiety as the children from restrictive homes, and they do not have the feeling that they have double-crossed the expectations and standards of those who have raised them. Most parents who do not have the sensitivity or courage to share openly with their children either conservative or liberal sexual values, do not ask too many personal questions of their youngsters, leaving them, by trial and error, to find their own way. The one tacit expectation is, "Don't get involved in pregnancy."

As will be more fully explored in the concluding chapter, there is also developing in contemporary religion an ethical viewpoint which admits the possibility of moral premarital coitus, and growing numbers of young adults are able to distinguish the issues and participate in intimacy without guilt. For many religious people virginity is no longer considered, in and of itself, a theological virtue. The question no longer is "to bed or not to bed?" It is "to become or not to become?" In other words, one can become a better, or more whole, person through responsible risks in interpersonal encounter. The religious issue is thus one of chastity. "Are my motives, intentions, and sensitivity to the other as pure as can reasonably be expected, insofar as I am aware of them?" This, after all, is the level of meaning which is more personal and significant to our lives than the abstract categories of ethics and the prohibitions which form neat theories more applicable to things than to human beings. The old morality which thought of chastity as cleanliness, as opposed to the dirtiness of coitus, today makes no contribution toward a healthy understanding of sexuality.

Today, chastity means acting with integrity. Virginity is the absence of a physical event which may or may not involve chastity. The point is that a virgin or a nonvirgin ought to be chaste—this is the essence of the single standard of sexual behavior. This quality makes a difference in how we look at ourselves. It provides us with the strength of self-respect which enables us to learn from, rather than be crushed by, whatever unanticipated painful experiences we may have, so that if the path of "going all the way" is chosen, we will not end in a dark pit of remorse, but will discover a highlight in the fascinating journey of becoming.

CHAPTER 7

Better Safe Than Sorry

T HE DAY IS NOT TOO DISTANT IN
America when mutual consent will be the only legal require-
ment of civil law governing sexual behavior and when contraceptives will be available to all who desire them regardless
of marital status. If present constitutional guarantees cannot be construed to protect the human right of sexual freedom to every citizen, then a movement must be initiated to
add a section to the Bill of Rights which will explicitly in-
clude sexual intimacy as an indispensable element of the right
to the pursuit of happiness. Even the conservatives of organized religion will be unable to suffocate the indignant and
insistent cries of the populace for such a sane social development. It may require the time of one more generation, since,
underneath the supposed moral reasons of those who oppose
such change, exists a deep jealousy and resentment because
healthy sensuality and intimacy were denied them in their day.
It is not easy to weep for what was missed and rejoice in the
joys of the young.

The perfidious charge against the unmarried is that, given
easy access to contraceptives, they will indulge in rampant
promiscuity and cause the nation to collapse with moral decay. How little confidence parents have in their children! Perhaps, also, parents are annoyed or threatened because they
now must assume greater responsibility for shaping the sexual
values of their children instead of foolishly relying upon the
deterrent of the fear of pregnancy. There should be serious
concern on the part of parents, educators, and religious lead-

ers, for we are dealing with a sexual revolution which will change the shape of interpersonal relationships, but we do not yet have clear evidence of things to come. Unfortunately, as in many controversial issues, the communication media give undue attention to the scandalous and the sensational, and, concerning sexual morality, the voices of reaction are heard while the progressives remain cautiously silent or write anonymously or under pseudonyms.

Access to reliable and convenient contraceptives *will* increase the incidence of premarital intimacy, but such relationships will *not* be promiscuous. Young adults, exploring the essence of one another in the wonder of sex are sensitive rather than cynical, caring rather than designing, and enter into close relationships with an honesty and an intensity that is a tribute to the human race. Should they be deprived of an intimacy that can contribute to their learning and growth? Is it moral for society to oppose such relationships that can prevent tragedy: forced marriages, ruined careers, the birth of the unwanted? Surely, we are confused and immoral when we deny contraceptives to the unmarried. Physicians, gynecologists especially, are caught in the middle of this transitional dilemma. They see the desperate need for their help, but either due to their own conservatism or primitive state laws, many hesitate to provide the information and the means which will prevent conception. It is, however, not the duty of physicians to force their moral standards upon others; rather, it is their professional obligation to provide medically reliable contraceptives to every patient who requests such services. Those who do so, and those who rise up angrily against antiquated civil and cultural prohibitions are owed a debt of gratitude. The time is overdue for the establishment of birth control clinics near every college and university in the country, as well as rural and inner-city clinics to serve all who walk in the door. Parents who allow their daughters to go off to work in cities or to college campuses without at least contraceptive information are moral cowards. Since postadolescent children are encouraged to make their own moral decisions, they have a right to birth control material without their parents' permission.

As for those young adults who are not of the character or sensitivity already alluded to, their need for contraceptive knowledge and means is imperative. Where the double standard is strong, where girls are exploited by boys and men, where ignorance prevails, this is where promiscuity is greatest and where birth control must be made available. Where there is not enlightened, responsible, and gentle standards for man-woman relationships, the war between the sexes is waged on a primitive level, whereby men and women abuse each other for immature satisfactions. This is promiscuity. And it is the promiscuous who need contraceptives the most! Promiscuous persons may use contraceptives—indeed it is hoped that they will—but widespread availability of conception-preventing drugs, chemicals, and implements will not in itself cause people to misuse sexual relationships.

Perhaps the contrary is true. Among the responsible who treasure their involvements, there are only so many simultaneous intimate relationships which can be satisfying. Intimacy involves the expenditure of tremendous psychic energy and time, and since there are so many other involvements and responsibilities in life besides the sexual, it is highly improbable that many people will take on more relationships than they want or need. Contraceptives will help a selected number of relationships last longer with deeper satisfaction and diminish the necessity to seek a greater number of partners. This result may also hold true for those who may be called promiscuous. If such persons are able to satisfy their physical and psychological needs, then they may be more inclined to limit their sexual searching and pay more attention to other nonsexual needs. Though all of this is speculation, it seems more reasonable than the anxious speculation that contraception for the unmarried will lead to an increase in promiscuity.

Contraceptives and Romance   Although the battle for nationwide availability of contraception is large, the primary tactical battle for responsible sexual freedom remains to persuade youth to *use*, not merely to know about, the contraceptives made available. There exist widespread ideas that contraceptives are unromantic and that premeditation ruins sex. For generations, the creed of the brave romantics has been, "Love conquers all; what will be will be." Anyone who believes that today with reference to premarital coitus without contraceptives is tempting fate. Other false notions also prevail: to have sex without safeguards is more pleasant; to plan beforehand is dirty. These notions had some validity in the age before the pill and in the era preceding the changing attitudes toward sex. There was a time when no "nice" girl would "do it," and when she did, it was proof of "love." Then, the diaphragm was the most reliable method. A diaphragm necessitates preparation and conscious decision, involves some inconvenience, interrupts spontaneity, and requires a service of measurement and prescription from doctors who often accommodate only reputable married people. There is, of course, also the condom, more easily available but inconvenient to the male and unreliable for the inexperienced. These contraceptives are greatly overshadowed by the pill and the intrauterine device (IUD), both of which will soon be replaced by the "morning-after pill" and other convenient drugs administered monthly and even yearly. Since there are excellent publications available explaining the types and merits of various contraceptives, it is unnecessary to duplicate this information here. Suffice it to say that every young man and woman should be aware of the inadequacies of condoms, and that no woman, under any circumstances, should use someone else's diaphragm or pills. Diaphragms must be fitted, and pills are drugs which necessitate prescription by a physician who will also conduct periodic checkups of his patient. Science is still dealing with hormones which react differently on each individual and which can be dangerous for persons with certain medical conditions. It is in the best interest of every woman using the pill and certain other contraceptives to remain under the care of her prescribing physician.

The central point is that there is no excuse for any woman to participate in coitus without dependable contraceptive security. Never leave it to the man who tells you he is taking care of it! For he will either depend upon a condom or plan on withdrawing his penis just before ejaculation, a method which, especially for the inexperienced, is far from dependable. Although we may wonder why male-dominated science concentrates primarily on altering female reproductive capability, the situation remains that women have the basic responsibility for not conceiving. Someday there will be drugs and chemicals which men may use to render themselves temporarily sterile, but, for the moment, we are dealing with a situation where only the woman has the means to prevent conception to a reliable degree.

These means should be used. They afford a woman protection and do not interfere with the emotional momentum on any given occasion. But let us face squarely the issue of spontaneity. Coitus does not just happen. We want it to happen long before the opportunity occurs. If a woman inserts her diaphragm before an interesting date, aware of her desires, she is using good sense. Or, better yet, if she is taking the pill conscientiously, she is prepared beforehand to make a decision for coitus without the worry of pregnancy. Such planning is honest and permits a greater degree of enjoyment. To put it another way, any young woman who cannot come to terms with her physical desires or needs, or who rejects the possibility of premarital coitus, must either have the courage to say "no" firmly, or experience the guilt of moral irresponsibility.

Young men share the same responsibility. If they seize fully upon the intensity of an emotional moment without ascertaining whether the woman is contraceptively prepared, they share fully in the consequences. No woman who becomes pregnant is solely at fault, and her partner must be held liable for either a follow-through in marriage or for financial and psychological support. Men sometimes face the risk that the woman may *want* to become pregnant as a means to marriage. Women face the same risk when they trust men to provide contraception, for some men have the corresponding desire to become fathers or to prove their "masculinity" by impregnating a woman. Thus, this entire question of motivation for contraception can become quite complicated psychologically. Any young person who thinks love is "free" has a lot to consider!

As consistently suggested in the preceding chapters, no intimate encounter is more worthwhile than the planned one, which has a basis in affection, understanding, and mutual consideration. Spontaneity in lovemaking is indeed an exciting and incomparable experience, but should not culminate in coitus without contraception. The pill, and the new substitutes are ideal for unplanned sexual enjoyment. Even if other methods are used, however, one will have greater pleasure and benefit from coitus when honestly premeditated, eagerly anticipated, and free of the possibility of pregnancy.

Menstruation and Coitus   Although this book is not a sex or marriage manual, it should be mentioned that there is a time in the ovulation cycle when contraception is not necessary, a time seldom talked about; this is the period of menstruation. We are not referring to the so-called safe period which the rhythm method of contraception relies upon, for this is a technique which requires careful attention and has inconveniences and a definite margin of error. Menstrual coitus is a time when pregnancy becomes less probable, especially if the boy also uses this occasion to experiment with the condom. What is being suggested is that the young woman who does not have a diaphragm or who is not on the pill but who would like to plan with her boyfriend a time to try coitus, might well consider the last half of the menstrual period as an appropriate time. It should be noted that unless the woman has a regular cycle with an average three- to five-day period the risk of pregnancy is increased.

In the future, relatively few couples will be deprived of reliable contraceptives and will not have to use the menstrual period to experience coitus. This "method" is mentioned, however, for what it teaches us about sexuality. It is very important for young men and women to have healthy, positive attitudes toward menstruation. Otherwise, it remains an insidious blockage in marital communication and communion. Before puberty both boys and girls should be knowledgeable about the facts of the ovulation cycle and the period of menstruation. Even more importantly, right attitudes about intimacy during this period should also be established so that man-woman relationships will not be distorted by taboos and old wives' tales. Sexually enlightened adults enjoy coitus during menstruation. Many people today accept menstruation casually, but it still remains a psychological phenomenon which causes enough uneasiness among enough people to be a problem. For countless generations women have been considered "unclean" during this time, and it is still common for people to think of the menstrual flow as the discharge of something foul or dirty, a "waste" product akin to urine or feces. Consequently, there are still women who consider their period as "the curse" when in actuality it is a wondrous blessing. Menstruation is merely the body's method of preparing for an impregnated ovum, and when this does not occur, fluids and substances, along with fresh blood, are released to prepare the woman for her next opportunity for pregnancy. While it may be said that the menstrual fluid is wasted, it should be considered a surplus material rather than a waste material. Girls should be proud of their menstrual flow—it is, after all, that which makes them a woman—and boys should be respectful of it rather than afraid of it or repelled by it.

Unfortunately, there are some girls who unconsciously feel dirty and who go through psychological contortions as well as some physical discomfort during their periods, while others will recognize within themselves heightened feelings of sensuality during menstruation. This is because they are almost completely safe from pregnancy, have more sensitive vaginal walls, and also need demonstrativeness from their boyfriends as evidence that they are desired. The man has no reason to be apprehensive about menstrual coitus, but if there is some hesitancy, a condom may initially be used until both partners accept comfortably the desirability of intimacy under this condition. Both men and women must cope positively with menstruation—the sooner, the better.

Choice of Contraceptives   Even if this book attempted to describe the types of contraceptives available, it would be outdated soon after publication. Any woman who wants a reliable contraceptive can do better than rely upon either the male condom or upon jellies, foams, or suppositories. Cervical caps and diaphragms are more reliable, and hormone pills or injections even better. The important point to be re-emphasized is that a competent physician or birth control clinic should be consulted in order to obtain the most effective, psychologically acceptable, and medically safe prescription for the individual concerned.

In the field of sexology, there are new discoveries to be

made and more illuminating hypotheses to be offered, but the values which will remain relevant are responsibility and sensitivity of men and women to bring out the best in each other.

Neither Safe Nor Sorry   As medical science works diligently to reduce even further the minimal risks of the various pills, it seems as if the promise of sexual utopia is near fulfillment. However, it is important to remember that immunization against venereal diseases has not yet been achieved. We still lack adequate forms of protection against the infectious bacteria of the various venereal diseases—diseases which can develop in all persons, regardless of sex, race, and educational and social status. Venereal disease is mentioned here not as a deterrent to sexual relations, but as factual recognition of a possible "side effect" of intimacy. Also, it is most important to realize that this is a *health* problem and not a *moral* problem. There is apparently an alarming increase in the incidence of venereal disease in this country, especially in the *fifteen* to *nineteen* age bracket. Some moralists seem almost delighted with these statistics, which can be used as a simplistic case against the enjoyment of sex. Fortunately, this inane prejudice is not common, and there is a renewed and sustained national effort to eradicate both gonorrhea and syphilis, communicable diseases which are a serious public health menace. But the eradication of these dread diseases cannot be accomplished by scientists alone, for the cooperation of every community and every infected person is indispensable. What cannot be emphasized enough is the absurdity of connecting shame or immorality with venereal disease. There was a time when mental illness was the most shameful thing that could happen to a person. Now, most people have the good sense to recognize its symptoms and seek therapy as soon as possible. Individuals who contract venereal disease must help bury the cultural taboo surrounding the subject and have the intelligence to recognize it as a medical problem.

So it comes to this, there is no absolute safety in intimacy. Yet, in what other sphere of life is it reasonable to expect such a guarantee? Responsibility only demands that we have knowledge of the probable consequences of our decisions; it does not require us to freeze with inaction, afraid to take risks which, according to our scale of values, we conscientiously judge as worthwhile for our lives. Though some diseases and some contraceptive side effects may yet plague us, we can, while science seeks to eradicate them, bear these trials with justifiable pride. We can be proud of the honesty to admit that we need the acceptance of our whole selves; the flesh as well as the spirit; of the sensual and emotional as well as the rational and intellectual. Although we are living on the edge of new relationships, we know enough to realize the dangers involved, but also the wonder of becoming and the sense of fulfillment achieved by sensitive uninhibited intimacy.

CHAPTER 8

Being Different

I F THERE IS ANY MANIFESTA-
tion of traditional, socially approved, sexual behavior which
should cause us seriously to question our moral presuppositions, it is our shocking and degrading treatment of the
homosexual, especially the male homosexual. Reason and
friendliness suddenly take the shape of insanity when confronted with even the thought of the homosexual. "If one of
those queers even so much as looks at me, I'll hit him," is
the brave statement of the uninformed. Since a few police-
men occasionally indulge in this sport for sheer sadistic satisfaction, it is no wonder that so many people think any
homosexual deserves inhuman treatment for the sake of the
public interest. The harassment, persecution, and social
ostracism of homosexuals are so severe that the more sensitive
will submit to blackmail or even choose suicide to prevent
exposure.

Why this irrational crusade against homosexuality? Not
surprisingly, it is given an aura of justification by primitive
religious prejudice. In our culture, the influential religion is
Christianity, and the Christian reading of its Jewish heritage
has propagated the "truth" that it is "natural" for man and
woman to complement each other's sexuality, and the purpose of this God-ordained relationship is procreation. Ortho-
dox Jewish and Christian theologies are being hard pressed
by the contemporary population explosion and the sexual
revolution which make the injunction to "be fruitful and
multiply" a quaint anachronism. The ancient wisdom, ex-

pressed in the powerful symbolism and eloquent mythology of the creation stories, is subject to radical revision. The mark of viable religion is not its tenacity to tradition, but its ability to promote and adjust to man's psychological growth and sociopolitical change. To assert dogmatically that the only "natural" sexual relationship is between man and woman is to ignore the fact that homosexuality is part of the story of man and that it can be a contemporary option for a healthy and satisfying relational life. In "common sense" terms, we ought to accept the fact that millions of men and women in this country need and desire sexual intimacy with persons of their own sex. We are obliged to question our right to deny them this relationship.

The Oddity of Men Against Men   Though the crusade against homosexuality is reinforced by archaic religious prejudices, religion alone cannot be blamed for this obsessive persecution. The primary cause has more to do with the male image of manhood, an image which is cultivated by a multiplicity of factors. The reason the Jewish and Christian theologies cannot bear the primary burden of blame is that these systems are male-centered and tend to promote the self-interest of men at the expense of women. It is the male homosexual, however, who is persecuted, while the female homosexual receives scant attention and little concern. Why? The male homosexuals do not support the male-dominated system. They threaten the security of other men, and they usually have a comfortable relationship with women, causing jealousy and anxiety on the part of other men.

The causes of homosexuality are complex and will continue to be the subject of research and debate. In the meantime, however, the realization that revulsion and hostility toward the homosexual are an emotional deviation as intense or neurotic as the sexual deviation itself, should cause us to cease our persecution of those who are not heterosexuals.

What Threat to the Social Order? The theological categories and religious prejudices which form the basis for legal statutes against homosexuality cannot be constitutionally justified. If a particular religion or denomination condemns this practice, then homosexual or heterosexual behavior becomes a matter of conscience for the individual who is a member of such a religious group. But in our pluralistic society the stand of one religion should not be forced upon all citizens through civil law. Fortunately, in addition to the various national, regional, and campus organizations of homosexuals which are striving for the eradication of these unjust laws, there are national religious bodies which are supporting the civil rights of homosexuals. The contemporary scene is encouraging in this respect, even though there is a long way to go before establishing the universal sexual right of mutual consent, including relationships within the same sex. It is ironic that the tyranny of social conformity wants the sexual deprivation and impoverishment of everyone who is not involved in a monogamous heterosexual union. Our traditional social expectation is both psychologically unhealthy and morally hypocritical.

Homosexuality poses no threat to the stability of the social order; on the contrary, it may even contribute to "the sane society." Is it not preferable for persons to seek a satisfying relationship with one of their own rather than to inflict torture upon themselves and marital misery upon others? Is it not better for women who would otherwise be destined to unbearable loneliness to know the comfort of intimate friendship with another woman? Homosexuals who understand and accept themselves can live as happily as anyone else and can be valuable contributors to society.

Cultural Brainwashing But isn't homosexuality an emotional sickness? According to some psychiatrists, it is. Supposedly, the enlightened approach to homosexuality is to see it, not as a sin, but as a form of neurosis. But this approach merely exchanges a sacred dogma for a secular dogma. Certainly, some people who are neurotic or psychotic may also be homosexuals, but the vast majority of such people with emotional problems are heterosexuals! Are we then to draw the valid but untrue syllogism that *heterosexuality* is evidence of mental illness? Of course not! Let us remember that the medical profession not long ago did nothing to eradicate the harmful belief that "excessive" masturbation caused insanity. Since many people under institutional or private treatment had a high incidence of masturbation it was erroneously thought that there was a causal connection between this act and mental disturbance. An act which may be considered a symptom of a rigid or fragmented personality may have a totally different meaning for an integrated personality. About all that can be said with any certainty is that homosexuality is an emotional illness for those persons who do not want to be homosexuals but who engage in it compulsively and have no control over its impulses. Only this type of person who admits his problem and who wants to change can be helped by psychotherapy.

Our society's concern for the homosexual is sincere but misguided. Operating under the assumption that only those sexual acts which end in coitus are "normal," we zealously seek to save the homosexual from his "perversion." It is about time we let the homosexual speak for himself. It is time for us to stop creating sickness in homosexuals, pressuring some into bizarre, defiant behavior by our cruel and repressive actions against them. With the same dignity accorded to every human being, and with the same degree of sexual freedom all of us may someday have, those who are homosexuals for neurotic reasons will increasingly recognize their own difficulties and seek appropriate therapy. We shall all be better off for such reasonableness. Sick patterns of homosexuality parallel sick patterns of heterosexuality, and the concern should be how to guide all people into healing rather than destructive relationships.

Not for Kicks   What has been said thus far hopefully establishes a positive approach to the phenomenon of homosexuality. This is not to say, however, that one ought to experiment with this practice. We really do not understand the factors which shape the development of a homophile (a lover of the same sex), and just as we should be careful in the use of hormones and drugs, so too should we be wary of prescribing for ourselves a homosexual experience. The implication is not that we should worry about any adolescent homosexual experiences we may have had. Group masturbation or mutual masturbation among members of the same sex, for example, does not mean that the participants are homosexuals. It is unfortunate that some people who have had such experiences harbor the secret fear that they are sexually abnormal and allow needless shame and anxiety to becloud their self-image.

Young adults, however, ought not to try homosexuality "just for kicks." There is the danger that, in the attempt to be sophisticated in sexual matters, they will not carefully consider the possible negative consequences of such an encounter. The same kind of self-knowledge and consideration of the other which applies to heterosexual intimacy also applies to responsible homosexual acts.

There is always the possibility that those who are tempted to try a homosexual episode will be unable to absorb the experience with any benefit. It is possible to be haunted for life with feelings of self-doubt concerning the ability to relate to the opposite sex. Even more disastrous is the possibility that the person who has a personality or relational problem but has had an initially enjoyable homosexual episode, will too easily settle for what seems to be the path to greater physical pleasure and psychological comfort, thereby prematurely and permanently destroying his potential for a satisfying heterosexual life. This is *not* to say that, once having a serious homosexual affair, an individual cannot develop a firm heterosexual pattern of behavior. But no one should take adult homosexual experimentation lightly. The experience may also prove to be very unpleasant, causing unexpected psychological trauma which can prevent full sexual enjoyment in marriage.

If a person has had an enjoyable homosexual experience, he may come through the episode with positive feelings and with no psychological harm whatsoever. But how about his partner? Granted, it is beyond the individual's control to guarantee how anyone else is going to react to any sexual experience. But does the one who is comfortable with the experience know his partner reasonably well to feel confident that he has not caused an unfortunate, possibly tragic, chain of events in the other person's life? What may be "kicks" or "education" for one may be destructive for the other.

Homosexuality does involve some legal and social risks which must be considered, especially if one's interest in homosexuality stems primarily from curiosity or the desire to please an older respected person. Although police officers are now less often invading the bedroom and the men's (ladies') room we still have with us the barbaric persecution and prosecution of homosexuals. The degradation of a police station booking and the scandal created by news media can demolish the character of the strongest of persons. If such entanglements with the protectors of the public can be avoided, there still remains the risk of social ostracism if someone is labeled a homosexual. The word has an amazing way of getting around. As incredible as it seems, there are men and women who have never had a homosexual experience, but who, because of stereotyped traits, are thought to be homosexual and treated accordingly. Choice of profession or marriage partner can be severely curtailed once the supposed homosexual has been put through the gossip mill. In a society as intolerant of harmless differences as is ours, experimentation with homosexuality still carries a very high price tag.

If You Are a Homophile   But what if a person thinks he is a homophile? Perhaps he has either tried and enjoyed a homosexual experience, or is obsessed with the fantasy and finds himself being aroused erotically by persons of the same sex. What if he thinks he is not merely curious about this variation in sex stimulation but that his love feelings seem to be predominately directed homosexually? What should he do?

First of all, he should neither hide in a corner nor jump out a window. There are, it is estimated, millions of people in this country who share his situation, and he is not alone. He is not a freak and not a criminal. He is himself and he has as much potential for a creative and satisfying life as any heterosexual. If he is young he stands a better chance of being accepted and of having a chance for self-actualization than homophiles of the past. There are at least three things he can do to help himself: be sure of his facts, avoid perilous situations, and be knowledgeable about the homosexual world.

He should talk to someone who is knowledgeable and understanding of homosexuality. Obviously, if he has the kind of parents, counselors, or clergyman whom he can trust and have an open, mutually respectful relationship, then, by all means, such persons are his best initial sources for help. The reason for exploring his feelings with a mature person first is that he may have some misinformation or misunderstandings about homosexuality. What he thinks or feels may be appropriate for his age or experience, and he may be jumping to unwarranted judgments and conclusions. If he thinks he is unusual or different, he owes it to himself to test his opinions against the wisdom of someone else with greater learning and experience. If he has no one with whom he feels he can have a confidential and sympathetic hearing, then he should read the best books on the subject he can obtain. Ultimately, no one can tell such a person with absolute certainty that he will or will not choose homosexuality as his primary pattern of sexual relationship. It is difficult, if he is not self-supporting, to go first to a psychotherapist, but, if there are mental health clinics in his area, he should walk in the door, tell his story to the interviewer, and let the clinic work on obtaining constructive cooperation from his parents. Young adults should not worry about the therapist trying to remake them against their will, because the therapist will try to help them make the most creative adjustment possible and will assist them in avoiding associated emotional difficulties. Any young person who thinks he has homosexual problems or a homophile personality should not be afraid or too proud to seek competent counsel as soon as possible.

People who are in an active, aggressive homosexual stage can help to advance the cause of all homosexuals: Stay away from young boys or girls. They should not be youth group leaders or teachers in segregated groups of their preference. Or, if they do assume these positions, they must have the self-discipline and the integrity not to initiate younger persons into the practice. Parents have every right to expect the teachers of their children to be protective and not expose them to potentially traumatic episodes. This holds true for both homosexuals and heterosexuals. The privileged position of leader or teacher is based on trust, protecting those under their care, and not taking advantage of their immaturity or emotional weakness. True, as far as homosexuality is concerned, children should learn, as part of their sex education, the facts of homosexuality and the calm techniques for rejecting homosexual advances. But this is almost a taboo subject, and nothing pushes the social panic button quicker than the cry of "child molester!" Given the reality of this social situation, there is no surer sign that a person's homosexuality is neurotic than his attempt to seduce young people. If there is any one factor which accounts for the hysteria about homosexuality and the ferocity of its persecution, it is this fear on the part of parents. This fear is indiscriminating, for seeking out uninitiated youngsters is not characteristic of the homophile. There is a kind of sexual deviant, the pedophile, who seeks sex play with children, and this type of personality is definitely in need of therapeutic help. To tempt younger boys or girls is to court personal disaster and to set back the just cause of the mature homosexual. If any person is determined to explore the homosexual pattern for his life, then he should seek other adult homosexuals. Today, this is easier than it has ever been due to the increasing openness and organization of homosexuals. The young person who recognizes homosexual desires should subscribe to the literature, join associations, and continually ask himself whether or not what he reads, hears, sees, and feels is really for him. If it is, if he understands and accepts it, he will not be forced into either extreme shameful secrecy or demeaning exaggerated behavior. He will instead find his place in the sun.

Relating to Homophiles   The overwhelming majority of men and women, those who orient their lust-love to persons of the opposite sex, ought to bear in mind two principles in dealing with homosexuals. First, if homosexuality is an emotional illness for some, then they should be accorded the same degree of understanding and compassion extended to a person with another type of psychological difficulty. Second, if homosexuality is a preferred way of life for some, we ought to grant such persons the human right of a behavior which does not harm us. The better we can come to terms with the homophile, the better we will understand our own inner selves.

CHAPTER 9

Parents and Lovers

Whatever the curses invoked or the legal punishments threatened against extramarital intimacy, it seems that increasing numbers of married partners are, with mutual conscientious consent, seeking a fuller life in extramarital relationships. These spouses who share similar desires, needs, and values beyond the satisfaction and benefits available in their monogamous commitment are usually labeled neurotic, perverse, unhappy, or worse. Those who hold to traditional exclusive monogamy find it impossible to believe that a husband or wife can be "shared" without destructive or tragic effect upon the marriage. This conviction is more a reflection of cultural conservatism than in accord with the responsible freedom of persons. Certainly there are innumerable couples who are devoted to one another, whose happiness is contained within their marriage, and who never think seriously of an intimate or extramarital relationship. But should it be necessary for such people to condemn others who have a different attitude and understanding of marriage and interpersonal relationships? It is time for this question to be asked openly, and it is time for the answers to be faced squarely. For it could be that the emotional reaction against the moral extension of sexual freedom reflects the uncertainties and anxieties of the conservatives more than the alleged immorality of the innovators.

"Adultery" is the catchall invective which makes the transgressors shameful. It is also the escape clause for the cynical sophisticates who use it as grounds for divorce and the gateway to serial polygamy. So-called adultery, as a reason for divorce, is nothing more than an excuse for terminating an unwanted alliance. This is so even among those who sincerely consider adulterous affairs as a break in trust and a betrayal of vows. To be sure, such feelings are understandable. What the sincerely religious often choose to ignore, however, are the ethical obligations of forgiveness and compassion. And, with a self-righteousness, they play the part of the martyr and rush into divorce. Adultery *may* be symptomatic of a troubled marriage, but of itself it should never be sufficient reason for the breakup of a marriage!

At this point you are probably wondering about the reasons for this discussion of extramarital intimacy and adultery addressed to unmarried young adults. There are three reasons. The first reason is that you had a father and a mother. Quite possibly there were times when you were mystified by some of the tensions between your own parents. Retrospectively, through a consideration of this issue, you may be able to put your family past and present in a more helpful perspective. Marriage and parenthood are not easy or simple responsibilities and children should not be naïve in judging parents or shallow in recognizing the qualities of quiet heroism in their fathers and mothers.

Second, you may possibly become a lover to a married person and ought to realize some of your responsibilities and the potentially destructive effects. While in the opinion of some the definition of adultery does not cover the unmarried partner, the participation in an adulterous alliance involves constant moral questioning and unwanted consequences for both parties.

Third, you may someday be married yourself and the time for reflection upon the realities of marriage is *now* while you are single. Hopefully you will not be shocked, crushed, or outrageously jealous when your spouse evidences interest in another person of the opposite sex.

Extramarital Intimacy and Adultery

Let us briefly consider the terms extramarital intimacy and adultery. Adultery by definition refers to an extramarital relationship which involves coitus. In most states it is an illicit act, and traditionally from a religious point of view it is considered immoral. As it is popularly used, "adultery" carries with it moral judgment and censure. A better term for adultery is extramarital intimacy—*an intimacy which may or may not involve coitus.* The question for married couples to face is, "Do we allow each other to have close personal relationships beyond our marital union?" This is a more creative concern than the usual anxious worry, "Would I be able to forgive my husband if he had an affair?" However, instead of assuming only the male to be the offender, it is more truthful to recognize the extramarital needs and desires of both men and women. Adultery and virginity are social controls. Historically they had definite social values relating to a framework of social, economic, and family values. However, not only have social, economic, and tribal conditions changed, but the equality of woman has been fortunately actualized, the psychological dimensions of relationships understood, and the scientific control of pregnancy placed within the determination of each couple. The fact remains that today we require a more enlightened development of interpersonal ethics and more reasonable civil laws governing marriage, divorce, and sexual behavior.

The discussion of virginity in Chapter 6 reveals the absurdity of the preoccupation with the technicality of penile-vaginal activity. If this supposed virtue of virginity is now merely a moral hangover, then it follows that the supposed vice of adultery is also a judgment or attitude with no relevance to our times. Again, then, the question which puts your sex values and attitudes to the ultimate test is, "When you marry will you voluntarily allow your spouse the freedom to enjoy the private company of another without jealousy and without worry as to the degree of intimacy involved?"

The Positive Aspects of Extramarital Intimacy

The values or benefits of a nonexclusive, nonpossessive marriage can be summarized in a general proposition: No one person can indefinitely and completely fulfill the needs, satisfy the desires, and enrich the interests of the marriage partner. For intellectual, emotional, and esthetic reasons extramarital intimacy relationships are often desirable and worthwhile. All men and women have such relationships in subtle and socially defined ways: The cocktail party or the beer blast are occasions in which we are thrown into carefree contact with other men and women; our formative childhood and adolescent years encourage the development of social abilities; single adults are urged to enjoy many dating partners and to enrich life with varied friendships. Then, all of a sudden, you are expected to find that one right mate and to live forevermore in marital bliss. This expectation is sentimental and unrealistic. Marriage can be of greater social significance and of greater worth to the individuals when we can admit the restrictive and limited aspects of the monogamous union.

Intellectually we change and grow. Contrary to popular assumption, it is not necessary for your spouse to share your professional and avocational interests and pursuits. The ingredients of a creative marriage have not yet been successfully analyzed, and to attribute it to "compatibility" is only to beg the question. It is ridiculous to confine a world of curiosity, knowledge, and interests to two—man and wife. Women suffer from this restriction severely. Men have a very free life.

They may go to conferences, conventions out of town, have luncheon meetings, and are unrestricted in evening arrangements, social or professional. Women, however, unless they are extraordinarily willful and competent in their special interests, are confined to the world of children and other housewives. Children, housewifery, and community activities are obviously rewarding and worthwhile responsibilities and contacts, but they cannot possibly exhaust the creativity and ability of many women who must suffer their interpersonal deprivations in gracious silence. A far richer world should be unlocked for women, and the key to it is greater maturity on the part of men. In practical terms men should, on a regular basis, either tend to the home for an evening or pay for child care to allow the wife a degree of integrity or freedom which enables her to go out without childish anxiety on the part of the husband. For example, is it wrong if a wife goes out with a male friend to a cultural or educational event in which the husband has no interest? Should not the husband rejoice that his wife is having a happy experience and is fulfilling herself as a person? And of course the same liberty should be allowed the man—an open and honest liberty which spares him the demeaning all too common practice of lying to his wife about his evening activities.

Let us be frank. From an exclusively monogamous point of view there are dangers in this freedom for interpersonal relationships, for it is possible that the spouse may develop a friendship-love for the companion causing jealousy in his spouse. (See Chapter 3.) Jealousy is a reflection of possessiveness and self-insecurity. Incredibly, we take it as a mark of true love or devotion, and often convince ourselves that this jealousy is a compliment to the desirability of the other. Jealousy in adolescence can be expected and is understandable. But one should grow beyond vulnerability to it.

Emotional Reasons   In all probability young adults will

undertake marriage with the romantic notion that they are perfect complements to their spouses. This assumption will sooner or later be unmasked as a delusion. As discussed elsewhere, monogamous marriage with its course of trials, challenges, and joys, is one of the primary, most satisfying, most rewarding stages of life. Nevertheless each person will do well to enter this relationship with the premise that he cannot at all times enrich and fulfill the emotional or psychological needs of his partner. All of us have our moods, our inadequacies, and our transitional growth periods, and consequently, there may be times when we will yearn for someone else to set a different pace or tone to our inner feelings. It may be that we will want to respond with empathy-love to someone who seems to need a relational encounter with us. Traditionally, the "for worse" conditions of the marriage vow, direct us to suffer through these times and lock our loyalties solidly within the one-to-one marital union. Is this reasonable? Is it human? Is it absolutely necessary to keep a marriage intact? There are reasons to believe that this is not so. In the course of growing up we are taught to reach out to others, and to open ourselves in trust to another when we or the other needs the balm of comfort, warmth, and affection. Why must the same style of living be abruptly halted with marriage? Every person has a very complex emotional or inner life and no one person, however treasured and loved, will be able to satisfy all the other's interpersonal needs. In the many relationships of our lives we do not expect to be all things to all men. There will, then, be times when a spouse has a deep friendship with another and this should be understood and not taken as a threat.

Esthetic Reasons   We feel lust-love until we are dead. As long as our senses function we derive pleasure from simply being in the presence of a person we consider attractive. Just because people get married and get older does not mean they no longer have the need to touch, to embrace, to feel, to caress other friends of the opposite sex for whom they feel affection. For people to be ashamed of their feelings of lust is a major tragedy of life. After all, if the world contains infinite wonders which we are encouraged to appreciate, should we not appreciate an attractive person who moves with grace and inspires us with the desire to be near him? Human beings come in all shapes and sizes with infinite variety of personalities and even colors. This magnificent multiplicity could be happily enjoyed in moral extramarital relationships. Monogamous marriage should not hinder such enjoyment. On the contrary, the exclusiveness and possessiveness of marriage is one of the prime causes of the silent warfare of most marriages. Obviously, there will remain countless numbers of married partners who will never desire extramarital intimacy. But the preference of such persons need not determine the pattern of married life for everyone.

The intellectual, emotional, and esthetic reasons for extramarital intimacy, involving the corresponding love-dimensions of friendship-love, empathy-love, and lust-love, are not, of course, simple reasons, for they are usually mixed with either or both of the others. Nevertheless, they are aspects of living which lead to greater self-realization and a more beautiful life for all, and it is time for the traditional view of marriage to be broadened in order to accommodate these deep-seated extramarital needs.

Negative Aspects of Extramarital Intimacy

Life and humans are much too complex for simple solutions and simple understanding. There are also potential dangers in, and drawbacks to, extramarital intimacy which must be considered. These involve escape from healthy marital tensions, the limitations of financial resources, the neglect of children, and poor communication between partners.

Escaping Healthy Marital Tensions As you read the previous sections on the positive aspects of extramarital intimacy, it is to be hoped that the thought occurred to you that people searching for such satisfaction and pleasure may be like little children obsessed with having a surplus of lolly-pops. Adults, after all, have the primary responsibilities of a home and family and should have the sense and self-control not to dash off into extramarital affairs every time something goes wrong, or they have a mood. Most marriages break up for the basic reason that the partners are self-centered and without self-discipline or moral courage.

Tension and conflict are inevitable components of any marriage. It is an awesome challenge to blend into a creative union two particular and peculiar persons. The danger in extramarital freedom is that one or both spouses will indulge in self-pity when problems occur and will too readily expend psychic energy and time looking for a "security-blanket relationship" outside the marriage. Such behavior is not easy to take or to forgive. Hurts and resentments sink deeply and often permanently into the relationship. A marriage is like a tender young plant which must be nurtured with great care and attention. When too many vital ingredients are siphoned off, the plant withers instead of blooming into its potential strength and beauty. The maturation time for each marital plant will vary, but it usually involves several years—years in which children may make additional demands upon the resources of the marital ground. In other words, tend to your family garden for your primary and sustaining nourishment.

The Limitations of Finances The popular assumption that poverty holds husband and wife together is no testimony to the virtue of poverty. It is closer to the truth to realize that the less money available the less there is left to spend on things other than family indebtedness. On the other hand, greater income and more flexible job schedules on the executive and managerial levels leave more time and money for extramarital interests. The truth is that the relatively wealthy have the option of greater sexual freedom and the sophistication to be properly discreet. The poor also have their methods of extramarital sexual excursions, methods which vary from subculture to subculture.

The majority of people fall into a vast middle category with neither the advantages of the well-to-do nor the disadvantages of the materially deprived. The average family has to be careful of its expenditures in order to maintain its conventional material comfort and usually has to plan for the expense of recreation. A night out, even to a movie, can be a fairly expensive proposition. Therefore, money spent by either the husband or the wife in extramarital pursuits can deprive the couple of shared experiences in recreational, athletic, or cultural events. Where money is tight it should be shared in a fair manner to provide some modicum of fun for both partners. It is necessary, then, that this matter be discussed by husband and wife in order to avoid resentments and not to jeopardize the total financial base of the family.

Neglect of Children   The proper care of children also involves money. But beyond this is the time invested in enjoying and knowing one's children. To be positively related to one's children is one of the most profound joys and privileges of life. Such a relationship is an achievement not guaranteed merely by the fact of biological parenthood. Consider the many functions and roles of parents: their respective jobs, their community involvements, their care for the house and planning for the future, and their daily attention to the needs and wants of the children. Unfortunately, it is often the children who get short-changed when parents have extramarital sexual interests. This is not always true, but parents have limitations to their physical and psychic energy, and it is a temptation to let the children exist apart from active and creative involvement in total family endeavors. Thus, when children are young and impressionable, parents should be on the alert to keep their extramarital involvements from causing their children to fail to enjoy a rich family life where they can grow to their fullest potential.

A Matter of Shared Values The critical challenge of marriage is communication. Coitus, when delightful and satisfying, can reflect communication at its deepest level of communion. When unsatisfying, it is often a reflection of a marriage in which there is conversation without communication. Communication obviously involves the nonverbal and nonrational forms of interpersonal exchange as well as the verbal and the logical. Herein lies a potential danger. The serious difficulties of marriages in which only one partner has convictions of extramarital sexual liberty are obvious and have been previously discussed. However, even in situations where both partners appear to share the same ideas, there may be unarticulated angers, jealousies, and resentments. One may change convictions after marriage without admitting it, or the feelings of one or both may not be correlated with conscious or expressed ideas. Indeed, the chance of two mature people with similar values of sex freedom marrying each other is probably rare. It is therefore a matter of degree, with always some negative feelings involved. Also there will be times when one partner will derive great help or comfort from an extramarital friend which may be resented by the other partner. Who can plumb the full depth of another's emotional dimensions? For that matter, who really understands that much about himself? Thus, extramarital relationships may ruin more marriages than they will enrich.

It is possible that in the future, as premarital sexual freedoms are incorporated into and accepted by society, couples will, in effect, live with each other for a period of time before they undertake the commitment of marriage. Hopefully, teenage marriages will decrease, unwed parenthood will decline significantly, and the advent of the first child will be a planned event. As premarital patterns move in this direction many more people will have experience in nonexclusive, nonpossessive intimate relationships and the transition to marriage will be less traumatic and more of a contribution to the wholeness of being.

Starry Eyes and Wishful Thinking   Any consideration of the practical dangers involved in extramarital intimacy must also admit the possibility of one of the partners "falling in love." There is a tendency for all people, at some time in their marriage, to wonder what their lives would have been like if they had married someone else. There is also a desire for most married persons, as they get older, to feel once more the sheer exhilaration of new love, and this can happen even after twenty-five years of satisfying wedlock. The vast majority of people do manage to contain these feelings within the bounds of innocent fantasy and social propriety. It is surprising that more couples do not part amicably after the children have left the roost, and perhaps more would do so if financial considerations and social customs permitted it.

There are other couples, however, in which at least one partner, in exploring the path of extramarital relationships, stumbles upon a romantic encounter with another person which sends him or her reeling. This can happen for many, many different reasons. It may be, for example, that the married couple has moved much further apart than they realized; it may be that this someone else has opened up new worlds of experience more significant than the married person had ever realized possible; it may be that this someone else simply meets more deep needs than his spouse ever satisfied; it may be that the married person, settled into a fairly mature "marriage of convenience," is suddenly brought alive by the extramarital relationship. Whatever the reasons, such topsy-turvy experiences can happen—and that's when all emotional hell can break loose. The possibility of this happening is increased when a married person becomes involved with another who is single, divorced and without children, or widowed. If you are an unmarried young or not-so-young adult, you should be especially aware of this potential consequence of an intimate relationship with a married person.

The basic reason why a married-nonmarried intimacy relationship is so unpredictable is that it is a more powerful one-to-one involvement. After all, the nonmarried (this word is used because it covers the single, divorced, and widowed) do not have the responsibilities toward a spouse to attend to, and they tend to be more demanding, perhaps even possessive, of the married lover: They tend, for various reasons, to seek a more total involvement. In response to this, the married person may feel a greater degree of obligation, and may even need the feeling of being wanted. Complicated? It certainly can be! If a married person creates for himself this kind of situation, and does not intend to separate from or divorce his spouse, then it is his obligation not to lead his lover on, and to disengage to a friendship-love plateau as gently, patiently, and lovingly as he is able. (Remember, by the way, that this literary "he" also includes "she.")

If all of these interpersonal complications shake up your youthful "free love" philosophy, the aggravation is worthwhile. *Think now* and save yourself some painful mistakes later. We have not, for example, considered the possibility that "illegitimate" children can be produced in extramarital as easily as in premarital relationships, for it is assumed that married people know the wisdom of contraceptive protection.

But, consider starkly what the alternatives are for the married person who "falls in love" with another: Suffering great sadness with attempted dignity; bumbling around in escapist affairs; going through the problems of obtaining a divorce.

There are, in conclusion, guidelines to be offered those on both sides who may consider being participants in a married-nonmarried alliance. Married persons would do well to consider restricting their extramarital relationships to other married persons. Nonmarried persons ought to accept beforehand the diffuse involvement of a married lover and not expect total attention and commitment from the married partner who intends to remain married. Every extramarital relationship requires nonpossessiveness, and the person who cannot accept this reality is better off not becoming involved in the first place.

Monogamous Nonpromiscuous Pluralism

The old moralistic dichotomies are dead, or at least dying. True, there are vast numbers of people who are nostalgic for the simpler ethic of "either-or": either a virgin or a whore; either pure or a pig; either chaste or lascivious; either faithful or promiscuous, etc., etc. The new premarital sexual ethic in which your generation is pioneering must eventually be reflected in new postmarital patterns of sex conduct. Hypocrisy, deceit, shame, unhealthy guilt, and the vicious exploitation of sex will in the near future be drastically diminished in marital, as it is being lessened in premarital, relationships. Unfortunately, in the meantime many pioneers will suffer in this transitional period. No matter how mature and discreet couples may be, many will be accused of being "wife-swappers" and will pay a heavy price in community ostracism, even the loss of jobs, and possibly face criminal prosecution. But the day will indeed dawn when a sounder sex ethic of nonpromiscuous pluralism within monogamy will be widely accepted.

Changes in the rendering of traditional marriage vows will mark the turning point. The number of otherwise alert and sensitive people who have a vague desire to be wed "in the church" or "in the sight of God" but who do not reflect deeply upon the words and meanings of the ceremony is astonishing. Young adults who conscientiously hold libertarian sex ideals will have to reflect carefully upon the promise to *forsake* all others and keep themselves only unto each other so long as they both shall live. Do all couples really intend to promise this? These words require the type of monogamy exclusive of extramarital intimacy. Those about to marry should consider very closely the promises repeated routinely after the clergyman in order to know what they are saying, meaning, intending, and promising. Then one must do one's best to live up to it; otherwise that lovely religious ceremony will be one of the most flagrantly hypocritical acts of a lifetime.

The intention to commit yourself to one spouse for a lifetime is indeed a precious hope, an ultimate value, and a risk worth taking. There are dimensions of life with one spouse which are superior to all other alternatives: the companionship of shared living which deepens as the years pass; the knowledge of another which only a sustained relationship can produce; the innumerable delights of nurturing children if children are desired and conceived; the warm and encouraging support of the other through the challenges and trials of life; the comfortable tenderness and closeness which can never be qualitatively equaled in extramarital relationships, no matter how worthwhile.

Marriage can create a richer life provided the union is carefully considered, mutually desired, and not exclusive of life-affirming intimate relationships with others.

CHAPTER 10

Toward a Religious Framework for Ethical Intimacy

A LEGITIMATE QUESTION WHICH occurs to many adults today is, "What makes so many clergymen so libertarian on sexual issues?" This kind of question is sometimes asked with an implicit accusation: "You have sold out to secularism. We are inundated with all kinds of sexual stimulation in our society. We do our best to bring up children with solid traditional morals, and when we send them to you—on whom we depend in this crisis—you seem even more radical than the children. Moral decay has, alas, corroded even the church! We don't need any "new" morality, we need to renew the integrity of those values which have stood the test of time and which have enabled us to attain the social stability and goods which have blessed our lives." There is honest bewilderment because religion seems to have been dragged compliantly into the salacious world of sensuality, and, at that, dragged, as some people think, by the Playboy philosophy! Therefore, before we consider some of the guidelines for ethical interpersonal relationships, it may be worthwhile to sketch briefly some of the intellectual and social influences of the last quarter century which caused a reevaluation of the human situation. Three such broad influences can be identified as existentialism, situationism, and technocracy.

Following the global devastation of World War II, there burgeoned a movement in philosophy and psychology known as existentialism, a movement that permeated so many fields and all of the arts media that its meaning became as diffuse as the current overworked term, "psychedelic." The traumatic recognition of man's willingness to use his vast learning for incredible destruction left the thinkers and artists of western civilization in a state of brooding introspection. With courage they explored relentlessly the stark possibility that life is absurd and that human responsibility is a cruel illusion. Without submitting to their despair, however, they shaped an attitude for the survival of sanity, an attitude of defiant hopefulness, an attitude which proclaimed, "I exist and I shall be free of demonic ideologies."

European theologians, especially, were affected by the existentialist attitude, and began to tear apart the encrustations of tradition with the daring assumption that they were either going to find some foundation of belief and value on which to rebuild or admit honestly the superficiality of the superstructure of religion. In America, we know the results of that search as "situation ethics," a viewpoint which reveals the folly of fitting persons into legalistic strait jackets. In effect, this school of thought asserts that the act of a specific individual, given his total situation, cannot be judged as morally equivalent to what seems to be the same act committed by another person who is responding to a different life situation. The morality of an act depends not on abstract laws or rules or mores, but on the quality of a person's conscience and choice, given *his* unique circumstances. This approach to morality frightens most people, for it seems to be too relativistic and to undercut the social security of fixed laws. This situational ethic affirms the superiority of the individual's integrity over all moral codifications, and places radical responsibility for morality where it belongs: in each acting, choosing, self-realizing person. Phrased in a negative sense, it means that every human being has the right to error, even to serious error, and that, in exercising this right, he also runs the risk of paying consequences for his action.

In addition to intellectual influences there are vast sociological and technological changes which demand new patterns
of human response. We face not only the problem of finding
new answers to old questions, but also new phenomena for
which there is no history of trial and error to guide us. For
example, the pick-and-shovel labor market is near the vanish-
ing point, and, any immigrant or racial group that wants to
succeed economically now needs more than sweat and muscle.
This demand for sophisticated technical education is not being met by our educational system which was modeled on a
blue-collar versus professional economic base. We now need
millions of technicians for thousands of new kinds of jobs
which didn't even exist ten years ago. This means extended
training and education even for those who are not going into
graduate professional fields of learning. Thus, a sexual morality which served a rural and a pre-electronic and preautomated
society will require radical revisions in order to meet the
needs of young adults who must go through an extended
phase of premarital existence. In cities and on campuses across
the country, millions of single persons are fashioning for
themselves the social patterns and behavior they need to establish satisfying human contact: Intimacy which will soothe
their anxiety in the face of academic pressure and vocational
uncertainty; contact which allows the freedom and the pleasure of exploring and defining themselves as sexual beings.

New attitudes on the part of organized religion toward
sexual issues ought to be viewed, then, in the total context of
religion struggling to be relevant in a rapidly changing world.
Ecumenicity, civil rights, peace crusades: These involvements
are all manifestations of religion recognizing and remember-
ing that the welfare of the Family of Man is the central subject of its ministry. Even this assertion is an inadequate
abstraction. We seek a goal beyond all ideologies, systems,
and acquisitiveness. Our society is at a maturational phase of

integration and interrelationship, and, if it looks as if the social order is disintegrating, it is only because we are looking through the crack in the picture window rather than stepping over the threshold into the action.

Do We Need Religion for Ethics?   This is an important question every individual ought to come to terms with because it underlies many of our sexual blocks, personal and social. From a practical point of view, it is reasonable to say that our society cannot afford to wait for theological agreement among its religions before enacting sane and uniform civil codes. The best that we can hope for is consensus among experts in jurisprudence, sociology, and psychology as to what course of action will afford the greatest health and freedom to the individual, while at the same time protecting society from those acts which can be considered criminal. The revision and enactment of law, therefore, involves dialogue among appropriate disciplines and eventual political compromise. What is then permitted under law could still be forbidden as immoral by any particular religion which promoted different values for its adherents. Because society permits sexual freedom does not mean that the individual must exercise this liberty. On the other hand, disrespect for law and abuse of the law prevails when a substantial number of people, who feel they can exercise responsible sexual freedom in good conscience, are prevented from doing so because of outmoded, quasitheological prohibitions. Perhaps this is all that needs to be said: Namely, that as a practical matter, society can transcend the ethical demands of different theologies.

Every philosophy, worldview, and religion, whether theistic or humanistic, has some set of values to which given acts may be considered moral or immoral, good or bad, right or wrong. Some of these positions are more flexible than others. Christianity has judged harshly the so-called legalism of Judaism and has prided itself on its so-called spiritual freedom.

Yet, Christians over the centuries have solidified an approach to sex which has been repressive and rigid, an approach which is, finally and happily, breaking down. The movement of rebuilding in a modern context is known as "the new morality" or "situation ethics" previously mentioned. Actually, this morality is not so much new as it is a radical recovery of the daring and imaginative spirit of the New Testament. Its greatest contribution to the understanding of Christian ethics is an unmasking of the kind of Christian hypocrisy and shallowness which limits morality to sexual issues—as if one cannot be immoral in racism, militarism, or commercialism—and to confront the individual person with his responsibility for moral decisions in every act of life. It asks the ultimate question, "What is the moral quality of this choice, given the situation," rather than the sterile question, "What rule did I break?"

Following is an outline of a religious framework for ethical decision making which is compatible with bare essentials of both Judaism and Christianity and which also has a place for other religious persuasions. For the sake of discussion, let us give this framework a name: relationalism.

Relationalism What in life is most real to you? Or, to put it another way, what about life do you most value? It would be surprising if your answer does not involve some important relationship you either have or want to have. Reality is not merely our random bumping into things or our passive drifting through events. Our reality is *encounter* with things and persons. It is the meaning about and feeling toward these experiences of encounter which characterize us as being human. Relationship is life. Good relationships are essential to mental health. Right relationships are essential to moral action. When we are unhappy or despairing, why? Is it not because we are fragmented within ourselves, or alienated from our friends, or because we feel cut off from God, or Life, or whatever we may call the mysterious ground of our being?

The worldview of Jesus was stated with powerful simplicity in his response to the question concerning the Great Commandment; the answer: to love with all of our being, God, our neighbors, and ourselves. Out of this tridimensional reality, sensitively felt and honestly faced, moral behavior will follow. The Great Commandment is not a list of do's and don't's, it is a comprehensive relationship! This conviction was not, of course, original with Jesus; it was central to his Jewish faith and was shared by his religious contemporaries, even by those who conscientiously rejected the startling claims made about him by his disciples.

The search for the wholeness of this grand relationship takes many forms and is understood in many ways. What a relational ethic asks in determining the moral quality of any act is this: "Did the individual touch all of the bases?" Did he seek not only to satisfy himself, but to bring out the best in the other according to the highest values he knows? Each of us, through our religious traditions will understand differently the meaning of God and the demands of this transcendent creativity upon us, will have different degrees of knowledge concerning the needs of others, will have different degrees of insight and self-understanding. What matters is that we *feel* the claims made upon us by these life forces and that we take the risk to *decide* what course of action we ought to follow.

Admittedly, such committed choices are not easy. Sometimes we will have to choose one good over another. Sometimes the same act will take on a different meaning because the context for choice has changed. Sometimes we may have to risk blaspheming God, or suffering the rejection of friends, or staring over the brink of sanity. Only you can experience the context; only you can make the choice. Should you exercise your human right for premarital or extramarital freedom? Such choice for intimacy *can* be moral, but only *you* can risk the decision.

Suggested Reading

It is not to be assumed that the author is in complete agreement with the following books or articles. These few materials are selected from the many hundreds of publications available because they are straightforward, nontechnical, and relevant to the topic of each chapter.

GENERAL RESOURCES

The Encyclopedia of Sexual Behavior, edited by Albert Ellis and Albert Abarbanel (Hawthorn Books, Inc., 1961).

The 97 contributors to this ambitious two-volume work provide a "who's who in sexology." While the 109 articles vary in quality, all are interesting and readable, providing information on a wide range of subjects. Every library should have this set available on open shelves.

The Playboy Philosophy, a series of editorials by Hugh M. Hefner, available in four reprint booklets (50¢ each) from *Playboy,* 919 North Michigan Avenue, Chicago, Illinois 60611.

These 22 editorial installments by *Playboy* editor Hugh M. Hefner, spanning the issues from December 1962 through May 1964, constitute the most thorough and lucid arguments for sexological re-evaluation and reform ever presented in this country. Concerning the impact of the magazine itself, the author agrees with the evaluation of Dr. William H. Masters that *Playboy* is "the best available medium for sex education in America today" (*Playboy,* May 1968, p. 200).

Sexology, a monthly magazine edited by Isadore Rubin, Ph.D. For men and women who want their sex knowledge increased without benefit of *Playboy*'s entertainment, this publication is indispensable. *Sexology*, in layman's terms, covers every aspect of sex and sexuality imaginable and is of value to both young and older adults. Available at major newstands (readers should not be put off by the occasionally garish covers), it is also obtainable through subscription ($5.00 per year), from Sexology Magazine, 154 W. 14th Street, New York, New York 10011.

SIECUS Newsletter, quarterly publication of the Sex Information and Education Council of the United States.

The first issue was published in February 1965, a month after this multiprofessional group was organized to research and promote comprehensive sex education curricula and to establish "human sexuality as a health entity." Under the leadership of executive director Mary S. Caledrone, M.D., SIECUS is responsible for remarkable progress in broadening the scope of sex education and developing new programs. Subscription to this valuable educational resource, which also includes two new study guides per year and two annotated book, audio-visual, and curriculum program lists per year, is $4.50. Write to SIECUS Publications Office, 419 Park Avenue S., New York, New York 10016.

CHAPTER 1

Education for Love: The Wider Context of Sex Education

Peter A. Bertocci, *Sex, Love, and the Person* (Sheed & Ward, 1967).

Dr. Bertocci, professor of philosophy at Boston University, challenges the young adult to view the meanings of sex and love in the context of the "dynamics of value in personality." Facing all of the hard questions concerning premarital sexual experience, he presents a persuasive and comprehensive case for the reservation of such intimacy until marriage. Sex education is put in the broader perspective of personal growth and responsibility to family and community.

Albert Ellis, *The American Sexual Tragedy* (Grove Press, Inc., revised edition 1963, available in paperback).

A devastating analysis of American sex-love customs by an authority on sexual behavior who is unfortunately too often ignored because of his controversial stands. This book, which exposes the hypocrisies and absurdities of contemporary sexual mores, is worth reading because it will sharpen the reader's awareness of society's confused sexual expectations and force a clarification of the goals of sex education.

Robert Grimm, *Love and Sexuality* (Association Press, 1964).

Love and sexuality and the problems associated with these aspects of human existence are treated in the doctrinal context of Christian faith. It is a bold attempt to state the relevance of theological orthodoxy to contemporary man-woman relationships.

Richard F. Hettlinger, *Living with Sex: The Student's Dilemma* (The Seabury Press, Inc., 1966).

Richard Hettlinger, an experienced college chaplain and teacher, knows the sexual dilemmas of college students and empathizes with their search for new standards of interpersonal behavior. This book is very well written, never evasive, and is a valuable resource for campus discussions of the subject.

James A. Pike, *Teen-agers and Sex: A Guide for Parents* (Prentice-Hall, Inc., 1965).

The subtitle of this book reveals its importance. Recognizing that sex education by parents is "sex education at its best," the former Episcopal Bishop of California outlines for parents the issues and concerns they must deal with if they are to communicate in a positive, helpful manner with their children. Parents need help in educating themselves in this field if they are to provide adequate guidelines for their children, and this book is a great asset in this undertaking.

Helen E. Southard, *Sex Before Twenty* (E. P. Dutton & Co., Inc., 1967).

Writing out of counseling experience with thousands of high-school young people, Helen Southard answers with refreshing directness many of the basic questions about sex and dating asked by adolescents. The title is somewhat misleading in that the book could best be utilized with teenagers under seventeen. It is equally relevant to the concerns of girls and boys.

CHAPTER 2

The Shame of Shame

The author is indebted to the writings and teachings of a number of theologians and psychologists for his understanding and formulation of the concepts of shame, guilt, and sin. It would, however, serve no purpose to present here a bibliography of specialized books or inaccessible articles.

Nevertheless, readers who may want to pursue this subject further would be well advised to begin with the writings of O. Hobart Mowrer, who, as a research psychologist, therapist, and active churchman, has a comprehensive grasp of the concepts of guilt and sin coupled with the courage to criticize both religion and psychiatry for their weaknesses in helping persons come to terms effectively with these personal and interpersonal realities. Specifically, Dr. Mowrer's collection of papers and articles, *The New Group Therapy* (D. Van Nostrand Co., Inc., 1964, paperback) is recommended. See especially chapter twelve, "Transference and Scrupulosity as Reactions to Unresolved Guilt," pp. 144–180.

CHAPTER 3

Love and Love and Love

Erich Fromm, *The Art of Loving* (Harper & Row Publishers, 1956, available in paperback).

Holding love as the answer to human existence, Erich Fromm nevertheless shows how varied are the objects of love and how difficult it is to grow as a loving person. This classic analysis of love should be studied by parents as well as by young adults.

Paul E. Johnson, *Christian Love* (Abington-Cokesbury Press, 1951).
In terms of what it means to be a member of the family of God and also in the context of family living, Dr. Johnson sensitively delineates the meanings of love. He discusses not only education toward love for the individual, but also the necessity for structuring the social order to allow for the development of a world community.

Joshua Loth Liebman, *Peace of Mind* (Simon and Schuster, Inc., 1946).
This book of pastoral guidance by the late Rabbi Liebman integrates psychological insight with religious commitment. See especially chapter four, "Love or Perish," in which the dimensions of love are interrelated with self, neighbor, and God.

Gibson Winter, *Love and Conflict: The New Pattern in Family Life* (Doubleday & Company, Inc., 1958, available in paperback).
Sociological and technological changes have shaped the emergence of the modern family. Dr. Gibson discusses this phenomenon with clarity, and his analysis of loneliness and the need for intimacy is brilliant.

CHAPTER 4

Self-Enjoyment

Lester W. Dearborn, "Autoerotism" in *The Encyclopedia of Sexual Behavior*, Vol. I, pp. 204–215 (see *General Resources*).
This article is a knowledgeable and straightforward treatment of the subject, and succinctly covers all aspects of this activity. Reprints of the article may be obtained from Lester Dearborn, Marriage Counseling Service, Boston YMCA, 316 Huntington Avenue, Boston, Massachusetts 02115.

Masturbation, SIECUS Discussion Guide No. 3 (see *General Resources*).
It is worthy of note that this SIECUS Discussion Guide is not

attributed to an author, although a concluding editorial note credits board member Warren R. Johnson, Ed.D., as the originator of the manuscript. The other members of the SIECUS board requested so many qualifications and emendations "in the attempt to do justice to a variety of viewpoints" that the result is more general and cautious than it might have been. Nevertheless, the guide is sound and merits wide distribution among parents and sex educators.

CHAPTER 5

The Pleasures of Petting

Peter A. Bertocci, *Sex, Love, and the Person* (see suggested reading for Chapter 1).

See also Bertocci's earlier work, *The Human Venture in Sex, Love, and Marriage* (Association Press, 1949), in which he makes a case against petting (pp. 17–43).

Richard F. Hettlinger, *Living with Sex: The Student's Dilemma* (see suggested reading for Chapter 1), especially chapter two, "Everything But," pp. 143–149.

CHAPTER 6

Going All the Way

Robert R. Bell, *Premarital Sex in a Changing Society* (Prentice-Hall, Inc., 1966, available in paperback).

Utilizing the works of Alfred C. Kinsey, Ira L. Reiss, and many other sex and family life researchers, Robert Bell presents a summary of the sociological study of sexual behavior in American society. The book is a convenient reference for those who want objective information in this field.

Evelyn Millis Duvall, *Why Wait Till Marriage?* (Association Press, 1965).

This is a valuable book for high-school age boys and girls who should know explicitly the many traditional reasons for not participating in premarital sexual activity. The positive values in sexual restraint, in the context of responsibility for self, family, and society, are clearly presented.

Lester A. Kirkendall, *Premarital Intercourse and Interpersonal Relationships* (The Julian Press, Inc., 1961).

This detailed study of 668 premarital intercourse experiences reported by 200 college-level young men focuses upon the values and moral standards which shape the quality of interpersonal relationships. Chapter ten, "Integration of Sex into Interpersonal Relationships" (pp. 228–252), should be read by young adults, for in that concluding chapter, Kirkendall outlines eight sociocultural forces that appear to operate in such a way as to "make it very difficult, if not impossible, to expect relationships of strength and integrity to result particularly from the more casual use of premarital intercourse" (p. 229).

Ira L. Reiss, *Premarital Sexual Standards*, SIECUS Discussion Guide No. 5 (see *General Resources*).

Summarizing four major premarital sexual standards, Dr. Reiss views realistically the trend toward increasing permissiveness and explores several of the reasons for this social development.

CHAPTER 7

Better Safe Than Sorry

The best source for popular and up-to-date information concerning the types and effectiveness of various contraceptives is the major women's magazines. Hardly a month goes by when one of these publications does not have an article on the subject. It must also be stressed that before a woman makes her choice of a contraceptive device, drug, or chemical, she ought first to consult an understanding physician.

The subject of venereal disease can be handled straightforwardly and effectively through the use of the *Teacher's Handbook* on *Venereal Disease Education* by William F. Schwartz, published by The American Association for Health, Physical Education, and Recreation, a department of the National Education Association (1965). This *Handbook* is used in conjunction with an unusual *Student's Manual* using the method of programmed learning. Parents, whose adolescents do not have this subject included in the health courses of their schools, could use this program in home study with their children (eighth grade and up). The *Handbook* ($2.00) and the *Manual* ($1.00) may be ordered from NEA Publications—Sales, 1201 16th Street, N.W., Washington, D.C. 20036.

CHAPTER 8

Being Different

H. Kimball Jones, *Toward a Christian Understanding of the Homosexual* (Association Press, 1966).

A summary of types of homosexuality, traditional approaches of the Judeo-Christian tradition, with guidelines for positive action for Christian churches, this book is a step toward understanding, though not approval, of homosexuals.

Mark Freedman, "Homosexuality Among Women and Psychological Adjustment" in *The Ladder: A Lesbian Review* (January 1968).

A copy of this issue may be obtained from Daughters of Bilitis (see below). Dr. Freedman's comparative study of women homosexuals indicates that "homosexuality is not necessarily related to psychological disturbance." His work complements a similar study by Evelyn Hooker on homosexual men published in an anthology, *The Problem of Homosexuality in Modern Society*, edited by Hendrick M. Ruitenbeek (E. P. Dutton & Co., 1963). Freedman, with co-author Dr. Mildred Weiss, plans to publish a book within a year on the relationship between homosexuality and psychological health.

Morton T. Kelsey, "The Church and the Homosexual" in the *Journal of Religion and Health* (January 1968, volume 7, number I).

The Rev. Mr. Kelsey summarizes Biblical and traditional church approaches to homosexuality as well as several psychological perspectives on the subject. Convinced that homosexuality is not a moral matter, he calls the churches to work for the civil rights of homosexuals and to manifest the same pastoral responsibility for them as is accorded any other person. This issue may be obtained from the Academy of Religion and Mental Health, 16 East 34th Street, New York, New York 10016.

Isadore Rubin, *Homosexuality*, SIECUS Discussion Guide No. 2 (see *General Resources*).

A brief but informative response to several important and common questions concerning causes and incidence of homosexuality.

Homophile Organizations

Though membership in such associations is apparently restricted to persons 21 years of age or older, information, and possibly advice, may be obtained from Daughters of Bilitis, 1005 Market Street, Room 208, San Francisco, California 94103; and for men, The Mattachine Society, Inc., of New York, 1133 Broadway, New York, New York 10010.

Note the distinction between the words "homosexual" and "homophile." Though the author is of the opinion that "homophile" is more descriptive than "homosexual," it should be recognized that some homophile groups do not consider the terms synonymous and use "homophile" as an adjective and "homosexual" as a noun. How widespread this consensus is, the author does not know.

CHAPTER 9

Parents and Lovers

Robert A. Harper, "Extramarital Sex Relations" in *The Encyclopedia of Sexual Behavior*, Vol. I, pp. 384–391 (see *General Resources*).

After citing incidences and legal aspects pertaining to the subject, Robert Harper offers fourteen observations about the pros and cons of extramarital relations. He discusses as well the issue of extramarital petting in a presentation that is concise and to the point.

Toward a Quaker View of Sex (Friends Home Service Committee, 1964).

This "essay by a group of Friends" published in England, quickly became a center of controversy. The first edition was shortly withdrawn from circulation because of bold implications concerning extramarital intimacy. The revised edition, however, maintains the possibility that such relationships can be constructive (see pp. 24–25 and p. 45). This attempt to develop a creative approach to sexual morality is not to be taken as an official position of Friends.

CHAPTER 10

Toward a Religious Framework for Ethical Intimacy

Joseph F. Fletcher, *Moral Responsibility: Situation Ethics at Work* (Westminster Press, 1967, available in paperback).

Joseph Fletcher, professor of social ethics and an Episcopalian priest, is the author of the innovating work, *Situation Ethics: The New Morality* (Westminster Press, 1966, available in paperback). His latest book is a comprehensive defense of the situationist ethic of love. Using specific issues in sex, medicine, business, and economics, he illustrates how genuine moral freedom involves responsibility.

John A. T. Robinson, *Christian Morals Today* (Westminster Press, 1964, paperback).

These three lectures by the Bishop of Woolwich analyze the tensions between fixity and freedom, law and love, and authority and experience in the context of Christian ethics. This brief work is a basic primer of the "new morality."

Sex Education and the New Morality (The Child Study Association of America, 1967).

This volume consists of the deliberations of the 1966 Conference of the Child Study Association of America, a meeting devoted to a search for a meaningful sexual ethic. It is a fine example of an effort to come to grips with new trends in interpersonal relationships.

Sex and Morality (American publisher, Fortress Press, 1966).

Presented as a committee report to the British Council of Churches, this document is of interest because of its incorporation of the "new morality" approach. It examines various aspects of sexuality and, ultimately, the committee found itself unable to fulfill its commission to prepare a "case for abstinence from sexual intercourse before marriage and faithfulness within marriage" (p. 5). The report was received by the Council of Churches without acceptance.

Selected Bibliography of Books
Relating to Alternative Lifestyles
in Family Life and Interpersonal Relationships

Bartell, Gilbert, Group Sex (New York: Signet, 1972), paperback.
Cuber, John, and Peggy Harroff, Sex and the Significant Americans (Baltimore: Pelican, 1972), paperback.
Kirkendall, Lester, and Robert Whitehurst, The New Sexual Revolution (New York: Donald W. Brown, Inc., 1971), paperback.
Neubeck, Gerhard, Extramarital Relations (Englewood Cliffs, N.J.: Prentice-Hall, Inc., 1971), paperback.
O'Neil, Nena and George, Open Marriage (Philadelphia: M. Evans, Inc., 1972).
Otto, Herbert A., editor, The Family in Search of a Future (New York: Hawthorn Books, Inc., 1970), paperback.
Rimmer, Robert, Thursday My Love (New York: New American Library, 1972).

ADDITIONAL RECOMMENDED GENERAL SOURCES
Forum: The International Journal of Human Relations
Forum Subscription Service, 155 Allen Boulevard, Farmingdale, New York, New York 11735. Published monthly, $12.00 per year.
Sexual Behavior
Sexual Behavior Subscription Department, 1255 Portland Place, Boulder, Colorado 80302. Published monthly, $10.00 per year.